ADOLESCENTS' COMMUNICATION: DEVELOPMENT & DISORDERS

Nancy L. Boyce, M.S.   Vicki Lord Larson, Ph.D.

ISBN: 0-9610370-5-9
Library of Congress Catalog Card Number: 82- 84480

Design: Graphic Source
Printing: Career Development Center by adults with developmental disabilities

Thinking Ink
Publications

7021 West Lowes Creek Road
Eau Claire, Wisconsin 54701

Authors

Nancy McKinley (Boyce) has her master's degree in Communication Disorders. After working in a public school setting for a number of years, she joined the faculty at the University of Wisconsin-Eau Claire where her primary responsibility is to supervise students during their field experience. Her interest in language disordered adolescents was solidified during a 2 year consultantship with D.C. Everest Public Schools that focused on developing an assessment and intervention model for their junior/senior high school students. Ms. McKinley is also a certified trainer of **Instrumental Enrichment**, a curriculum designed to teach thinking skills to those past 10 years of age. She has given an extensive number of presentations on the topic of adolescents' communication and thinking skills at various agencies, schools and conventions.

Vicki Lord Larson holds her doctorate degree in Communication Disorders and has presented nationwide on topics pertaining to language development and disorders. Her audiences have appreciated her ability to integrate theory and application and to present her ideas clearly and concisely. Currently, Dr. Larson is on the faculty at the University of Wisconsin-Eau Claire. She has taught a variety of courses pertaining to all aspects of assessment and intervention with school age language disordered students. Dr. Larson has held numerous consultantships, the most recent being with the Division of Corrections working with young adults in the prison system identified as language disordered. She is also engaged in on-going communication research projects with adolescent students along with Ms. McKinley.

PREFACE

The intent of this publication is to provide a working manual
for educators concerned with developing oral communication
skills in adolescents. The authors do not intend this manual
to be a panacea on the topic of Adolescents' Communication. If
anything, it is a crude beginning. This manual is working
toward: (1) establishing effective and efficient assessment
and intervention strategies for older students with language
disorders; (2) integrating theoretical knowledge and practical
application; (3) encouraging active participation by the readers
to adapt the general principles to their specific job settings;
and (4) coordinating the available information from across the
related disciplines.

Many professional disciplines currently have research, theories,
tests, and materials that are applicable to the population discussed in this manual. It would be foolhardy for speech-language
pathologists to rely solely on the field of Communication Disorders
for their resources because current information is sparse and
there are vast amounts of knowledge in related disciplines. Some
of the information used in this manual comes from such diverse
journals as Journal of Research in Science Teaching, Harvard Educational Review, and Journal of Philosophy for Children. What the
authors have found is not a paucity of available data, but an
overwhelming amount of information housed in many different pro-
fessions. This manual is an attempt to bring about a wedding of
the available concepts along with integration of our own ideas.
We readily admit this may be a wedding of insufficiencies, yet it
is an attempt to sort out what is available and useful.

As professionals become more skilled in working with language
disordered adolescents and as more valid research is conducted,
we hope a stabilized partnership will result from speech-
language pathologists and contributors from other disciplines.

Communication is included in the title to emphasize the authors'
position on what they believe to be the ultimate goal for language disordered adolescents, namely to learn how to become effective oral communicators. Oral communication is a dynamic, ever-
changing, social process in which there is an interchange between
a speaker and a listener. During this communication process, the
speaker sorts, selects, and sends symbols through a medium such
that the listener can find within his/her own mind a meaning like
that intended by the speaker. Ineffective communicators may display speech or language pathologies, or both. However, for

purposes of this publication, language pathologies and the impact they have on communication are emphasized. Therefore, the reader will not find specific information on phonological disorders, fluency disorders, or voice disorders.

The authors chose speech-language pathologist to refer to members of the profession of Communication Disorders, since it is the professional title adopted by the National Office of the American Speech-Language-Hearing Association. The readers should note that, occasionally, specific reference is made to the speech-language pathologist. The authors did not intend that this manual be directed only toward members of this profession, but rather to those in all professional disciplines interested in serving adolescents with oral language disorders.

You will find the manual divided into six main sections. The first section, "Overview," addresses our society's expectations of adolescents and the concomitant problems that result when these expectations are not fulfilled. This section also provides an historical perspective on the concept of adolescence and encourages readers to explore their own attitudes toward this period of development. Professionals harboring primarily negative reactions toward adolescence may not be the educators most capable of eliciting optimal response from older students.

The second section is called "Philosophical Premises" and shares with the readers basic, underlying beliefs that the authors share and that influence the assessment and intervention processes they recommend later in the manual. This section also describes a delivery model to use with language disordered adolescents within a school setting and suggests criteria for entrance and dismissal from the caseload.

The third section, "Assessment," discusses the assessment process and provides strategies to determine if the problem is within the student, the educational system, or the environmental conditions. Assessment strategies for the student include the areas of case history, cognitive skills, language comprehension/listening, language production/conversational skills, and survival language skills. Questions regarding "What to Assess" and "How to Assess" are addressed. Formal instruments and informal procedures are listed for each assessment area. The assessment of the educational system is accomplished through the use of CALI: Curriculum Analysis - Language of Instruction, an instrument developed by the authors. The assessment of environmental conditions is accomplished through interviews and situational analysis. Activities to be completed by the readers are intertwined throughout "Assessment."

The fourth section, "Intervention," attempts to integrate the results from assessment and the intervention plan. By encouraging readers to "go back" and examine how questions were answered

v

in the "What to Assess" sections preceding "Intervention," they can design appropriate strategies for the student. Each major area (cognitive skills, language comprehension/listening, language production/conversational skills, and survival language skills) includes a discussion of general strategies for intervention, specific goals/strategies, and commercial programs/resources available. Intervention strategies are also suggested for the educational system and environmental conditions. Again, the reader is asked to complete activities following each subsection of "Intervention."

The "Glossary" is the fifth section, highlighting specialized vocabulary used within the manual as defined by the authors. The "Bibliography" section follows.

We have only begun research on the topic of adolescents with language disorders. We need to work together toward a greater understanding of their needs. In our attempt to successfully complete this endeavor, please share with us any ideas, premises, and strategies you wish. We welcome your correspondence.

Nancy McKinley (Boyce)

Vicki Lord Larson

ACKNOWLEDGMENTS

For the past five years, the authors have become increasingly interested in studying and implementing programs for older students with oral language/communication disorders. During these years, we have profited from our interactions with numerous people. Each of them has contributed to our current theoretical and/or clinical knowledge base.

Specifically, we wish to thank:

Elizabeth Rowe Godwin who was a co-author of our first manual and for two years a co-presenter in our junior/senior high workshops. Her creativity has had a direct impact upon our service delivery model and ideas for assessment and intervention.

Paul Hager, who has contributed greatly to the section on normal adolescence development by reviewing the literature and organizing the volumes of data in a systematic and concise fashion.

Nancy Meyer, Linda Schwartz, and Chris Winslow have willingly field tested and critiqued many of our ideas in this text in the public school setting and their constructive feedback has provided us with the necessary data to refine and modify our work, especially in its latter stages. We graciously acknowledge Ken Hobbs and the D. C. Everest Public Schools for the pioneering efforts they made in establishing criteria for entrance to the caseload.

A special note of thanks to Dr. Terrance Sheridan, Eau Claire Public Schools Assistant Superintendent and the students and their parents at DeLong Junior High School and South Junior High School for allowing us to tape and analyze adolescents' conversational styles.

For assistance in editing the manual, we wish to thank Karen Welch. For her countless hours in typing this manual, we are indebted to Beverly Rongholt. For our families and friends who tolerated our absence many evenings and weekends, thank you for being there when we returned home.

TABLE OF CONTENTS

OVERVIEW

EXPECTATIONS AND PROBLEMS AMONG ADOLESCENTS

I. INTRODUCTION

From our own personal histories, interactions with adolescents today, and clinical observations, certain expectations about how students in grades 7-12 should communicate have been built. There are always those outstanding students who are held up as models, and then a variety of adolescents who fall within a wide range of normalcy. Below that range lies a group of students with communication disorders who may be in the mainstream or receiving special educational services of some kind. These are the students who display problems in oral communication, speaking, and/or listening. Frequently, these same students also have deficits in their cognitive development. When oral communication and thinking skills are too far out of line with expectations of educators, parents and peers, problems arise.

II. EXPECTATIONS AND PROBLEMS

A. Cognition

1. Students are expected to be at the formal operational period; the problem is they have remained concrete operational thinkers.

2. Students are expected to observe, organize, and categorize data from an experience; the problem is they can bring "Chaos to Order."

3. Students are expected to identify problems, suggest possible causes and solutions, and predict consequences; the problem is they may not recognize the problem when it exists; if they do, they do not know how to develop alternative solutions.

4. Students are expected to put items and ideas into sequential order; the problem is they cannot sequence events and main ideas.

5. Students are expected to gather, select, and organize data on a given topic; the problem is they have no strategies for finding and selecting the data.

B. Language Comprehension/Listening

1. Students are expected to comprehend all linguistic features and structures; the problem is they are misunderstanding advanced syntactical forms.

2. Students are expected to listen to lectures, and to select main ideas and supporting details; the problem is they do not grasp the essential message of a lecture.

3. Students are expected to follow oral directions of three steps or more after listening to them one time; the problem is they do not realize that they were being given directions.

4. Students are expected to critically analyze other speakers; the problem is their judgments are arbitrary, illogical, and impulsive.

C. Language Production/Conversational Skills

1. Students are expected to use grammatically intact utterances; the problem is they use sentences that are fragmented and that do not convey their messages.

2. Students are expected to have a vocabulary capable of expressing ideas and experiences; the problem is they have word-finding problems as well as a high frequency of low informational words.

3. Students are expected upon request to give directions, make a report, explain a process, or express an opinion, and to do so with clarity and accuracy; the problem is they often leave their listeners confused.

4. Students are expected to get information or assistance by asking questions and to respond appropriately to questions asked of them; the problem is they may know what question or answer to give, but not how to do so tactfully.

5. Students are expected to produce language that is organized, coherent, and intelligible to their listeners; the problem is they use many false starts and verbal mazes.

6. Students are expected to follow adult conversational rules such as initiating conversation, maintaining a topic, indicating topic changes, and considering their listeners' awareness levels; the problem is they consistently violate the rules.

7. Students are expected to follow adult nonverbal communication rules such as using appropriate eye contact, maintaining appropriate personal space, and avoiding distracting gestures that distort the verbal message; the problem is they consistently violate the rules.

8. Students are expected to be effective listeners during conversation without displaying incorrect listening habits such as calling the subject dull, criticizing the speaker, or letting emotion-laden words get in the way; the problem is they have poor listening skills.

9. Students are expected to express their own attitudes, moods, and feelings and to disagree appropriately; the problem is their conversational speech is often abrasive.

D. Survival Language Skills

1. Students are expected to comprehend and use specialized phrases and vocabulary required for survival in our society; the problem is they do not have the necessary concepts and words needed in places such as banks, grocery stores, and employment agencies.

2. Students are expected by their peer groups to use the slang and jargon of the hour; the problem is they do not understand it or produce it appropriately, thus ostracizing them from the very groups they most desire to be members of.

III. SUMMARY

When examining the communication of adolescents, certain expectations are held by parents, teachers, and/or peers in the area of cognition, language comprehension/listening, language production/conversational skills, and survival language skills. When the behavior falls significantly below expectations, problems result. Given a cluster of problems due to oral communication and cognitive deficits, one begins to recognize adolescents with language disorders.

IV. <u>ACTIVITIES</u>

    A. List additional expectations that you or other educators in your agency hold for adolescents.

        1.

        2.

        3.

    B. List the corresponding problems that result when the expectations you listed above are not met.

        1.

        2.

        3.

    C. List any of the expectations cited by the authors that your agency does not hold for adolescents.

        1.

        2.

        3.

NORMAL ADOLESCENCE

I. INTRODUCTION

In Western society, adolescence is the transition period between childhood and adulthood. As a stage of development, adolescence is influenced by an interaction among physiological, sociological, and psychological events.

   A. <u>Physiologically</u>, adolescence is marked by biological sexual maturity.

   B. <u>Sociologically</u>, adolescence is viewed as the transition to independent, self-sufficient adulthood. Most societies use either <u>functional criteria</u> (e.g., ability to support oneself) or <u>status criteria</u> (e.g., voting rights) to mark the end of adolescence.

   C. <u>Psychologically</u>, adolescence is marked by that point at which one establishes independence (such as freedom from uni-lateral control and influence from both parents and peers.) An integration of self-concept occurs, resulting in a per-sonal sense of identity. Adolescence is also believed to be a time of accelerated cognitive growth as stated in <u>Compensa-tory Education in Early Adolescence</u> (1974), and it is during this developmental stage that we see the emergence of formal operational thought.

II. EXPECTATIONS

All of us have preconceived notions about adolescents, either due to memories of our own youth or our interactions with today's adolescents. These ideas influence our expectations about their behavior. It is important that we analyze when our judgments are subjectively rather than objectively based.

Write down your first reactions when you hear the word "adoles-cents."

   A.

   B.

   C.

   D.

   E.

5

III. THEORISTS

A number of theorists have contributed to our knowledge of adolescence.

A. Hall, S. (1904) pioneered modern scientific investigation of adolescence as a distinct and separate stage of human development.

B. Freud, A. (1948) wrote a book on the ego and the defense mechanism.

C. Eriksen, E. (1968) has researched adolescent personality development and concluded that one of the major developmental tasks in adolescence is the formation of an identity.

D. Mead, M. (1950) has studied adolescents from an intercultural perspective and found that not all cultures are stage oriented. Some cultures such as the Samoan society do not have a period of development called adolescence. They view the life cycles as a continuous, gradual process from birth to death.

E. Tanner, J. (1974) contributed to our knowledge of adolescent physical maturation.

F. Piaget, J. (1958) in his book entitled The Growth of Logical Thinking, discussed the content of the formal operational period of development. This cognitive period of development begins during early adolescence.

G. Kohlberg (1975) has devised a theory of moral development based on Piaget's cognitive developmental hierarchy.

IV. WESTERN SOCIETAL INFLUENCE

The transformation of America from a primarily rural, agragarian society to a primarily urban industrial society has greatly influenced our concept of adolescence.

A. Changing demands of an industrial society created three major social movements which transformed the idea of adolescent time span into a social reality:

1. Compulsory education laws

2. Child labor legislation

3. Special legal procedures for juveniles

B. Technological change is occurring at a logarithmic rate. Because society must change to accommodate technological advances, we find ourselves living in a society which is continually changing.

C. Current societal change has an impact on the behavior of the adolescent:

  1. Traditional values, skills, and standards seem increasingly irrelevant, weakening the ties between generations.

  2. The future seems increasingly uncertain and unpredictable -- more emphasis is placed on the present.

  3. Depersonalization of society makes it increasingly difficult to meet affectional needs.

D. The changing concept of adolescence is reflected in legislation granting 18-year olds full legal rights and responsibilities (26th Amendment).

E. Sociocultural dimensions influence our expectations of adolescence.

  1. Western society is stage-oriented, and adolescence is a creation of our society.

  2. Benedict (1976) cites three major areas of "discontinuity in the life cycle" in Western society:

    a. Responsible vs. nonresponsible behavior

    b. Dominance vs. submission

    c. Changing sexual roles

F. Not only is the social environment of adolescents changing, but the adolescents themselves are changing in terms of personality, physical, intellectual, and moral development.

V. PHYSICAL MATURATION

Physical development can be discussed in terms of:

A. Sexual maturity

B. Growth in height, muscular development, lung capacity, and heart size

C. Growth of the brain

D. Vocal characteristics (voice changes occur during adolescence, but are rather late in the developmental sequence (Tanner, 1974).)

1. The growth of the male larynx is accelerated due to the influence of testosterone (Tanner, 1974). The vocal folds increase in length and thicken, and the voice pitch drops about a full octave (Zemlin, 1968).

2. In females, the larynx grows at about the same rate during adolescence as it did throughout childhood (Zemlin, 1968). At the end of adolescence, the female voice pitch has normally dropped about two or three musical notes (Zemlin, 1968).

3. Males between the ages of 9 and 13 have a modal pitch of 220 with a range of 150-250. Between the ages of 14 and 16, they have a modal pitch of 180 with a range between 130 and 225. Between the ages of 17 and 18, they have a modal pitch of 130 with a range between 90 and 180. The adult male has a modal pitch of 115 with a range of 70-160 (Mueller, 1982).

4. Females between the ages of 9 and 13 have a modal pitch of 240 with a range of 170 to 300. Between the ages of 14 and 16, they have a modal pitch of 225 with a range of 160 through 290, and between the ages of 17 and 18, a modal pitch of 215 with a range between 150 and 280. Adult females have a modal pitch of approximately 200 with a range between 140 to 270 (Mueller, 1982).

5. Fundamental frequency is not fully established until age 25 for both sexes (Mueller, 1982). For more detailed information see Table 1 that follows:

Suggested Modal Pitch Level & Range By Age And Sex

At birth regardless of sex 500 Hz.

	MALE			FEMALE	
Age (Yr.)	Mode (Hz.)	Range (Hz.)	Age (Yr.)	Mode (Hz.)	Range (Hz.)
1-3	300	225-400	1-3	300	225-400
4-8	260	200-325	4-8	260	200-325
9-13	220	150-250	9-13	240	170-300
14-16	180	130-225	14-16	225	160-290
17-18	130	90-180	17-18	215	150-280
Adult	115	70-160	Adult	200	140-270

Table 1. Reprinted by permission from Mueller, P. 1982.

VI. MORAL DEVELOPMENT

    A. Kohlberg's Theory of Moral Development (1975)

        1. Moral stages form an invariant sequence of development.

        2. Moral development can terminate at any stage of development.

        3. Each stage is an organized system of thought.

        4. Individuals cannot understand moral reasoning more than one level above their predominant level of moral reasoning.

        5. Individuals are attracted to moral reasoning one stage above predominant level of moral reasoning.

        6. Stages are what Kohlberg refers to as "hierarchical integrations."

        7. Advancement through the stages of moral reasoning depends upon the interplay of three factors:

           a. Cognitive development

           b. Ability to role-take or emphathize

           c. Cognitive disequilibrium

    B. Stages of Moral Development (Kohlberg, 1975)

        1. The Preconventional Level involves a punishment/reward system.

           a. Stage 1 - Punishment - Obedience is defined by the person's judgments based on avoiding punishment or obtaining rewards.

           b. Stage 2 - Instrumental Relativist Orientation is determined by the person's judgments based upon reciprocal favors or fulfillment of needs.

        2. The Conventional Level involves social conformity.

           a. Stage 3 - Interpersonal Concordance is based on judgments determined by conformity to persons in authority.

           b. Stage 4 - Law and Order Orientation is based on judging or obeying laws and social rules.

3. The Postconventional Level involves humanistic concerns.

   a. Stage 5 - Social Contract Orientation is defined as judgments made on the basis of individual rights and standards that have been agreed upon by the whole society.

   b. Stage 6 - Universal Ethical Principle Orientation is defined as judgments made on the basis of consequence in accord with ethical principles such as justice and respect for human dignity.

C. Kohlberg's Theory Criticized

   1. Kohlberg's theory of moral development has been disputed recently by Siegal (1980) as having an invariant sequence for all six stages, particularly the early stages. Siegal (1980) proposed that Kohlberg's method relies too heavily on responses to moral dilemmas which are outside a subject's personal experiences. Nevertheless, Kohlberg's Stages 4 and 5 are useful in that they characterize types of moral reasoning in adolescence and adulthood.

   2. According to Gilligan (1982), Kohlberg's theory fails to consider the differences in stages of moral development between boys and girls during early adolescence. She concluded that young girls are different from young boys and do not adhere to the stages advocated by Kohlberg's Theory. Research still needs to be done on the differences, if any, between the sexes during middle to late adolescence.

VII. SUMMARY

In Western society, adolescence is a period of development between childhood and adulthood in which numerous physiological and psychological changes take place. Although at times the literature is vague and conflicting, it provides a vast array of ideas for further investigation. It is critical that readers be familiar with the available body of current literature on the normal development of this period if they are to assist those with disorders.

PHILOSOPHICAL PREMISES

I. INTRODUCTION

There are certain philosophical premises upon which services to older language disordered students (middle grades through junior/senior high) should rest. These premises are derived from research, theory, related literature, and clinical observations and experiences. The list of premises selected by the authors is not meant to be comprehensive, nor are items mutually exclusive. However, each item is considered critical to the ultimate success of providing services to older students who are language handicapped.

II. PHILOSOPHICAL PREMISES

A. Older students who are language handicapped have been neglected in the public schools by speech-language pathologists because:

1. Higher education neglected to train these professionals to work with older students.

   A survey conducted by Boyce, Godwin, Larson (1979) revealed that only 50% of the training institutions accredited by the Educational Training Board of the American Speech-Language-Hearing Association in Minnesota, Iowa, Wisconsin, Michigan, and Illinois have formal course work in language assessment and remediation of this population.

2. Professionals have been conditioned to believe that early intervention negates the need for later services. A Stanford Research Institute report, Compensatory Education in Early Adolescence (1974), noted that extensive educational efforts with some older pupils may be effective because some students experience accelerated cognitive development during adolescence.

3. Until recently we did not have to provide needed services to this population.

   With the passage of P.L. 94-142 (Education for all Handicapped Children's Act) and certain states mandating services (i.e., Wisconsin Statute 115) all handicapped students between 3-21 years are guaranteed a free appropriate education.

11

B. Materials, methods, and service delivery models traditionally applied to preschool and elementary students are not directly applicable to students in the middle grades through senior high school because:

1. The students are different. Brown (1978) stated that older handicapped students are different from younger students in their need for:

   a. Increased behavioral independence

   b. Increased mobility beyond the school setting

   c. Increased feelings of failure and consequent lowered self-esteem

2. There are changing variables within the educational system. Brown (1978) highlighted some of these:

   a. Secondary schools cease teaching the basic skills and assume they are mastered.

   b. Teachers assume the student is an independent learner.

   c. Students learn best through the lecture.

   d. Students must cope with a varied schedule of classes.

   e. Students have different teacher styles to learn to cope with.

   f. Junior/Senior high school students are being asked to make vocational decisions.

   g. Extracurricular activities within the school become increasingly important for social acceptance.

   h. The departmental administration of junior and and senior high schools is foreign to most speech-language pathologists at the elementary level; likewise speech-language pathologists may be foreign to the administrators and regular educators at this level.

3. The family/social system demands are different.

   a. There is less parental involvement in school and everyday life, but increased parental concern about achievement and post-high school planning.

12

b. There is increased peer pressure to conform
    (Brown, 1978).

C. Problem students may have severe basic skill deficits.

The National Youth Workers Conference in Washington, D.C.
(July, 1982) emphasized the growing evidence that many
students who have problems with drug and alcohol abuse
have underlying skill deficits. These deficits go
beyond reading and writing problems. There are problems
with speaking and particularly, listening skills. A re-
curring theme is that an increasingly higher percentage
of our youth fall into the category of being everyone's
problem but no one's responsibility. The schools find
programs for them too costly and feel they do not qualify
for P.L. 94-142 services; they have not committed a crime
serious enough to put them into the criminal justice
system, and they do not qualify for social services.

D. Speech-language pathologists must be knowledgeable of
    normal adolescent development as derived from profes-
    sional disciplines of psychology, linguistics, speech-
    communication, and English.

    1. Simon (1981) advocates a look at other professional
        journals for data on this age group.

    2. Various professional disciplines have contributed
        to our knowledge of normal cognitive-communication
        development (Inhelder and Piaget, 1958; Feuerstein,
        1980), moral development (Kohlberg, 1975), and
        language development (Loban, 1976; Poole, 1979;
        McCroskey, 1981).

    3. Knowledge of normal communication development is
        critical to determining the existence of a communi-
        cation disorder.

E. Whenever possible, assessment procedures should be
    derived from existing knowledge of normal adolescent
    development and should encompass both formal and infor-
    mal testing strategies.

    1. Emerick and Hatten (1979) discussed suggestions for
        guiding their work with adolescents. Among these
        suggestions is the notion of acquiring knowledge
        of normal adolescence.

    2. Miller (1981) discussed three different types of
        procedures:

a. Standardized tests or formal procedures

b. Developmental scales

c. Nonstandardized or informal procedures

Each of these procedures has its own particular application depending upon the client. Usually, more than one procedural type is required.

F. Intervention strategies must be developed jointly by the speech-language pathologist and language handicapped student.

1. Simon (1981) stated that the students should understand why they are working on a particular skill.

2. Alley & Deshler (1979) stated that students should be active participants in the learning process. Students need to develop alternative solutions to problems if they are to function adequately as adults.

G. Cognition and language interact, and each influences the other. Although numerous cognitive theories exist, the authors have primarily utilized the works of Inhelder and Piaget (1958) and Feuerstein (1980). These two theoretical positions are not completely compatible, nor are they necessarily incompatible.

H. Older students with language disorders should be taught strategies (see definition in the glossary) and not specific subject content for two reasons:

1. Speech-language pathologists are not tutors to the curriculum, but rather intervention facilitators.

2. Strategies allow students not only to meet immediate requirements, but to generalize these skills across various situations and settings.

III. SUMMARY

These eight philosophical premises are based upon research, theory, related literature, and our clinical observations and experiences. This list encompasses only general premises; it is assumed that readers would have additional, specific philosophical viewpoints unique to their particular settings.

IV. ACTIVITIES

A. List the philosophical premises unique to you in your job setting:

    1.

    2.

    3.

    4.

B. Which philosophical premises presented by the authors are not ones to which you could subscribe?

    1.

    2.

    3.

    Why?

DELIVERY MODEL

A DELIVERY MODEL FOR SERVICES

I. INTRODUCTION

Taking into account what is known about normal adolescents and utilizing the underlying philosophical premises, a model for serving adolescents with language disorders has been developed. The delivery model addresses the issue of how assessment and intervention services can be most effectively and efficiently implemented at the secondary level. The authors' proposed delivery model involves coordination of four elements: information dissemination; identification; evaluation and program planning; and intervention.

II. ELEMENTS OF THE DELIVERY MODEL

A. Information Dissemination

1. Why is it important that we disseminate information?

   a. It heightens awareness of language disorders in this population. In an unpublished survey of clinicians in Wisconsin by Boyce, Godwin, and Larson (1979), more than 50% of the responding speech-language pathologists stated that their colleagues were unaware of the range of services they could provide.

   b. It ensures appropriate referrals from individuals who work with the older language disordered student. Appropriate referrals, in turn, can lead to appropriate services.

2. What information needs to be disseminated?

   a. The interrelationship of communication skills with academic and social performance during adolescence needs to be discussed. The developmental nature of language and communication skills is critical information to disseminate, particularly pointing out that speaking and listening skills precede reading and writing skills. If a teenager is not yet intact with regard to the spoken language system, it is common for the written language system to also not be intact. Information presented by Johnson (1982) indicated that out of the 90 learning-disabled adults she evaluated, 68 had oral communication problems, over 80 had reading problems, and all of the adults had writing problems.

16

b. The expectations for speech-language-communication behavior for those past the age of 10 need to be identified.

c. The types of speech-language-communication problems that can exist among this population and the individuals who would thus need to be referred for assessment is necessary information to disseminate.

d. The options for delivering appropriate services to language disordered adolescents (see Section D of "A Delivery Model for Services") is critical information to share.

3. Who needs to receive information about our services?

a. Students with oral communication problems need the information. Established speech-language programs in junior/senior high schools report that self-referrals begin when students realize their peers are receiving valuable intervention for which they might also qualify.

b. "Regular" educators in the classroom need the information since they are often the people who identify the problems.

c. Guidance and vocational counselors could use the information to better serve their clients.

d. Special educators need to be aware of the information so that they can make appropriate referrals.

e. School administrators, particularly the building principal, and school board members need to receive the information to gain funding support for the delivery model. The importance of these individuals receiving and assimilating that information cannot be overemphasized. Unless the people who make program and staffing decisions are involved in recognizing the need for speech-language services for older students, these services can easily become one of the first cuts in the budget.

f. Medical personnel, particularly those who interact frequently with people in this age range, are important target people for this information.

g. Social service personnel, including those who work with the criminal justice system, need this information.

h. Parents, who have so much invested in their children -- past, present, and future -- <u>deserve</u> to receive this information!

B. <u>Identification</u>

1. Why is it important to identify students with suspected needs?

   a. It is mandated by P.L. 94-142 that appropriate services be provided for school-age students with language disorders.

   b. Time is limited! These students have a minimum number of years left before they are expected to assume a responsible position in the community and have basic survival skills.

2. Who will identify the students?

   a. Self-referrals can occur with the adolescent population. They are very aware when they "suffer" differences from their peers.

   b. Educators, administrators, special, and support staff members within the school may all help identify students.

   c. Social service personnel working closely with students outside the school may be first to identify a need.

   d. Youth worker staff members, such as social service personnel, are in an excellent position to identify needy students.

   e. Medical personnel can be extremely influential, especially in the case of disorders resulting from trauma or disease.

   f. Parents, who know their children better than anyone else, could identify a suspected problem.

3. How will identification of students be accomplished?

   a. An effective referral system is the best way to identify students. People cited in the previous section will have participated in information dissemination and thus will know when a referral is appropriate.

18

b. Mass screening is not recommended by the authors, even though mini-screening tests for adolescents have been developed (Prather, et al, 1981; Prather, et al, 1980). Time spent screening is not efficiently used at the secondary level.

c. Using an observational checklist, which can be returned to the speech-language pathologist, can keep the number of unnecessary referrals to a minimum. The following sample form created by the authors is based on a rating scale where "5" is the highest possible score and "1" is the lowest possible for each item. In addition, "NA" may be used to indicate "not applicable" or "no chance to observe." Twenty behaviors are checked in four major areas: cognition; language comprehension/listening; language production/conversational skills; and survival language skills. The highest possible overall score is 100 (20 items x 5 = 100) if all items are rated. School districts could establish predictive cut-off points for students needing additional services based on their particular population. A starting point of 50% could be used to indicate a significant oral communication deficit from the educator's perspective (e.g., 50 points out of 100 if all items are rated; 30 points out of 60 if 8 items are not rated).

SECONDARY LEVEL REFERRAL FORM: COMMUNICATION DISORDERS

Course or Specialty:_____   Educator:_____
Date Completed:_____   Total of All Ratings:_____

Using the following scale, mark the following statements regarding the communication behavior of
_____ in your classroom.
    (student)

5 -   Almost Always
4 -   Frequently
3 -   Sometimes ("50-50")
2 -   Infrequently
1 -   Almost Never
NA -   Not Applicable/no chance to observe

COGNITION

_____1.   The student recognizes problem situations.

_____2.   The student generates alternative solutions for problem situations.

_____3.   The student engages in inductive reasoning (i.e. "specific" to "general").

_____4.   The student engages in deduction reasoning (i.e. "general" to "specific").

_____5.   The student collects data, compares and contrasts that data, and generates
             hypotheses.

_____TOTAL

LANGUAGE COMPREHENSION/LISTENING

_____1.   The student indicates that he/she comprehends main ideas presented.

_____2.   The student follows a sequence of directions even if asked only once.

_____3.   The student identifies relevant supporting details and records them in a notebook
             and/or systematically retrieves them on request.

_____4.   The student uses critical listening skills such as detecting fact from opinion,
             evaluating a speaker's argument, and recognizing propaganda.

_____TOTAL

LANGUAGE PRODUCTION/CONVERSATIONAL SKILLS

_____1.   The student plans what he/she is going to say, sequences it in a logical way, and
             produces the resultant sentence(s) with few verbal mazes.

_____2.   The student uses grammatically intact sentences; sentence fragments are ap-
             propriate to the context (e.g. Student answers with a single word in response to a
             question such as, "Where is he going?")

_____3.   The student easily finds words to communicate as precisely and accurately as
             possible and avoids use of low informational words (e.g. "stuff", "things", "what-
             chamacallit")

20

Larson, V. and Boyce, N. © 1983

_____4. The student provides relevant and complete answers to questions.

_____5. The student interacts verbally with educators and other students, being considerate of their feelings, taking turns speaking and listening, and initiating and maintaining conversations.

_____6. The student displays normal voice characteristics with regard to pitch, volume, and quality (i.e. lack of chronic hoarseness, breathiness, etc.).

_____7. The student displays normal fluency characteristics (i.e. lack of word or syllable repetitions, prolongations of sounds, silent gaps within words).

_____TOTAL

SURVIVAL LANGUAGE

_____1. The student demonstrates comprehension of basic spatial and temporal concepts.

_____2. The student demonstrates the ability to obtain and keep a job with his/her present level of language/communication skills (i.e. Would you hire this student given the way he/she talks and listens?)

_____3. The student demonstrates sufficient language to cope with daily living situations such as job applications, shopping, using the telephone, interpreting signs and labels, etc.

_____4. The student uses figurative language acceptable to the peer group.

_____TOTAL

Cognition Total: _____
Language Comprehension/Listening Total   _____
Language Production/Conversational
Skills Total: _____
Survival Language Total: _____
TOTAL OF ALL RATINGS: _____/_____

I feel confident in this student's ability to independently function once his/her school experience is over. _____

If you rate this item "1" or "2", please comment on how the student's oral communication is contributing to the problem:_____

_____

_____

C. Evaluation and Program Planning

1. What is accomplished during evaluation and program planning?

   a. The existence of a communication disorder and the need for speech and language intervention services are determined.

   b. An individual education plan (IEP) that best meets the needs of the student evaluated is completed.

2. Who participates in evaluation and program planning?

   a. Appropriate professionals are appointed by the Local Education Agency (LEA) to participate in the evaluation (e.g., learning disabilities specialist, speech-language pathologist, school psychologist).

   b. The student who is being evaluated participates. By this point in their educational careers, students need to participate in planning their programming, and help to determine what is most critical to learn in the time remaining.

   c. The parents of the student evaluated participate. They also will have insight regarding what is most critical to learn in the time remaining. In order for communication skills taught at school to generalize to other situations, it is crucial for parents to be aware of their child's program plan and "own" some of the responsibility for implementing it.

   d. The intent of program planning is collectivity. A staple does not make a comprehensive, organized IEP. People cooperatively planning create the best individualized educational objectives.

D. Intervention

1. Why not use the traditional model we have already established?

   a. Removing junior and senior high school students from classrooms for 20 minutes twice a week disrupts time schedules.

   b. Walking in or out during a class period is one more way the language disordered student looks different from peers.

c. Speech-language pathologists keep themselves removed from the routine in the rest of the building. Developing relationships with other professional colleagues can become difficult.

d. Speech-language therapy can easily be viewed as punitive rather than beneficial. Students receive no credit for work that may be very difficult for them.

2. What kind of model would be more appropriate at the junior/senior high level?

a. Offering language intervention as a course for credit (e.g., ¼ credit/semester) is more appropriate. Students invest at least as much time and energy working on their communication skills as they do on other skills taught as courses for credit.

b. Giving a grade, or using a "Satisfactory-Fail" system, as other courses would, is more appropriate.

c. Utilizing the time blocks <u>as they are already established</u> in the school system (e.g., a 45-minute module) is more appropriate. Students are seen on a predictable established schedule, as in all other classes. In many cases, this may involve all five days of the school week.

d. Grouping students into small classrooms, with the exception of those few who truly need a 1-to-1 therapy setting, is more appropriate. In the majority of cases, students need to be grouped to facilitate group interaction processes.

e. Using a room that is located in an "acceptable" part of the school building according to peer dictates is more appropriate than conducting intervention in the "special education" wing of the school.

f. Working closely with other educators in the building to coordinate efforts during intervention is more appropriate than acting completely independently. Speech-language pathologists need to be aware of the curricula in which the students are involved and to help identify how oral language deficits are interfering with learning. At the same time, speech-language pathologists must be careful to not become a tutor to those curricula.

The emphasis needs to be on teaching compensatory strategies, not content.

g. Becoming a part of the "team" at school as much as possible is appropriate. This can be facilitated by attending faculty meetings, participating in after-school events, coaching, or providing faculty supervision for clubs, organizations, special projects.

h. Calling the intervention program "Communication Skills" or another similar name is more appropriate than calling it "speech" or "speech therapy." The latter label will not be appealing to the majority of adolescents.

III. SUMMARY

The proposed delivery model coordinates the elements of information dissemination, identification, evaluation and program planning, and intervention. The model is specifically designed to integrate normal adolescent development, expectations and problems among adolescents, and the authors' philosophical premises. The need to disseminate information about students who are "everyone's problem, but no one's responsibility," followed by identification and evaluation/program planning, is emphasized. Only then can appropriate intervention services begin.

IV. ACTIVITIES

A. Compare and contrast the implementation of the proposed delivery model in an urban vs. a rural setting.

	· RURAL	URBAN
Similarities:	1.	
	2.	
	3.	
	4.	
Differences:	1.	1.
	2.	2.
	3.	3.
	4.	4.

B. How would you adapt the proposed delivery model to best meet the needs of language disordered adolescents on your caseload?

1.

2.

3.

4.

CRITERIA FOR ENTRANCE AND DISMISSAL

I. INTRODUCTION

The authors hesitated to include a section on criteria for entrance and dismissal from speech-language intervention programs because of fear of its misuse or abuse. If you are rigid in applying these standards to your employment setting, there is a strong possibility that students who need help may not be serviced. These criteria are included only as guidelines to consider in generating your own criteria in your respective employment settings. They should be used in a flexible, thoughtful manner to insure that appropriate services be rendered to adolescents with speech-language disorders.

II. CRITERIA FOR ENTRANCE

A. It is suggested that adolescents with the following characteristics not qualify for speech-language intervention services:

   1. Students whose language problems result from the lack of desire rather than the inability to communicate within the school environment, and who are receiving appropriate services.

   2. Students whose language problems result from learning English as a second language and who are receiving appropriate services.

   3. Students whose communication problems simply reflect environmental, cultural, or dialectical influences.

   4. Students whose pragmatic systems are disordered, but who have intact phonological, morphological, syntactical, and semantic systems, and who are receiving appropriate services.

B. It is suggested that adolescents with the following characteristics do qualify for speech-language intervention services:

   1. Students who have a 50% or more discrepancy between actual and expected performance levels as determined by language comprehension/listening tests using formal instruments or informal procedures (minus two standard deviations on standardized tests).

2. Students who have a 50% or more discrepancy between actual and expected performance levels as determined by language production/conversational skills testing, using formal instruments or informal procedures (minus two standard deviations on standard tests).

3. Students who have insufficient language/communication skills to survive routine life experiences (e.g., money, time, space) as determined by basic life skills testing, using formal instruments or informal procedures (minus two standard deviations on standard tests).

C. It is suggested that examiners use judgment when determining whether students with the following characteristics qualify for speech-language intervention services:

1. Students who have a 20-50% discrepancy between actual and expected performance levels as determined by language comprehension/listening tests, using formal instruments or informal procedures (between one and two standard deviations on standardized tests).

2. Students who have a 20-50% discrepancy between actual and expected performance levels as determined by language production/conversational skills testing, using formal instruments or informal procedures (between one and two standard deviations on standardized tests).

3. Students who have language/communication skills to survive some routine life experiences but not others (e.g., money, time, space) as determined by basic life skills testing, using formal instruments or informal procedures (between one and two standard deviations on standardized tests).

D. Students who are in other categorical programs such as classrooms for the emotionally or behaviorally disturbed, those with learning disabilities, the educable mentally retarded, or the trainable mentally retarded do not automatically qualify for speech-language intervention services. Needs of these students are to be considered in light of the above suggested criteria.

III. CRITERIA FOR DISMISSAL FROM THE CASELOAD

A. It is suggested that adolescents who exhibit the following characteristics be dismissed from the caseload:

1. Students whose language comprehension and production skills have improved from a 50% discrepancy level to within a 20 to 25% discrepancy level as determined by

formal and informal testing procedures; this communication performance level must have been maintained for at least one year.

2. Students who have become disinterested in working on their language/communication skills and thus have made minimal progress during a three to six month span.

3. Students who exhibit a high incidence of absenteeism for no justified reason.

B. It is suggested that adolescents who exhibit the following characteristics be monitored prior to dismissal from the caseload:

1. Students whose language comprehension and production skills are within a 25 to 30% discrepancy level and who are using those skills inconsistently in school and at home.

2. Students who have only recently exhibited the behaviors described in III A, 2 and 3, thus resulting in a dramatic mismatch with past performance.

IV. SUMMARY

This section introduces criteria for entrance and dismissal from the caseload. The authors strongly recommend that the criteria be applied cautiously and with the appropriate modifications for your employment setting so that they help obtain appropriate speech-language services for adolescents.

V. ACTIVITIES

    A. Critique the authors' criteria for entrance and dismissal according to your employment setting.

        1. Strengths

            a.

            b.

            c.

            d.

        2. Weaknesses

            a.

            b.

            c.

            d.

    B. Add appropriate criteria for entrance to your caseload. What is your rationale for these additions?

        1.

        2.

        3.

        4.

    C. Delete inappropriate criteria for entrance to your case-load. What is your rationale for these deletions?

        1.

        2.

        3.

        4.

D. Add appropriate criteria for dismissal from your case-
    load. What is your rationale for these additions?

    1.

    2.

    3.

    4.

E. Delete inappropriate criteria for dismissal from your
    caseload. What is your rationale for these deletions?

    1.

    2.

    3.

    4.

F. What differences, if any, would cognitive deficits in
    the student make in your criterion for entrance or dis-
    missal?

    1.

    2.

    3.

    4.

ASSESSMENT

OVERVIEW OF THE ASSESSMENT PROCESS FOR ADOLESCENTS

I. INTRODUCTION

Initially, when approaching the assessment process, it is
important for the examiner to ask, "Where is the problem?"
and "Whom should we assess?" It is essential to ask and
answer these questions because the problem may not be with
the student. Rather, the problem may be within the educational or environmental systems. In the educational system,
the educator may be the problem, suffering from "dyspedagogia"
(i.e., the inability to teach). The problem may be within
the curriculum. The language concepts may be too advanced
for the student to comprehend or the curriculum may be dis-
organized. Within the environment, the problem may be with
the family and/or the peer group's attitudes, values, and
beliefs which impinge upon the student and affect performance. Both the educational and environmental systems must
be evaluated before concluding that the student has the problem. Figure 1 illustrates this more global approach to assessment of the adolescent.

II. GENERAL ASSESSMENT PRINCIPLES

Assessment strategies for evaluating the adolescent student
are discussed below from a general philosophical perspective. It is the authors' contention that these principles
should be considered and implemented to their fullest:

A. Determine the Purpose for Assessment

Determine exactly why you are assessing the student.
Is the purpose to screen the student to determine if
further assessment is warranted? Is the purpose to
determine the existence of a problem or the goals of
intervention, or to plan specific intervention procedures? These questions must be answered first in order
to determine the specific information needed and the
techniques to use in the assessment procedure (Bloom
and Lahey, 1978).

B. Acquire Knowledge About Adolescence

1. Acquire a working knowledge of the period of development called adolescence. Recognize that in Western
   society, adolescence is a transition period between
   childhood and adulthood.

31

FIGURE 1. OVERVIEW OF ASSESSMENT STRATEGIES

WHERE IS
THE PROBLEM?

ASSESSMENT
STRATEGIES

STUDENT

EDUCATIONAL
SYSTEM

ENVIRONMENTAL
CONDITIONS

WHAT

1. CASE HISTORY
2. COGNITIVE SKILLS
3. LANGUAGE COMPREHENSION
   / LISTENING
4. LANGUAGE PRODUCTION/
   CONVERSATIONAL SKILLS
5. SURVIVAL LANGUAGE SKILLS

1. LANGUAGE OF INSTRUCTION
2. CURRICULUM CONTENT

1. FAMILY
2. PEERS

HOW

1. INTERVIEWS
2. FORMAL TESTS
3. INFORMAL PROCEDURES

CALI:
CURRICULUM
ANALYSIS-LANGUAGE
OF INSTRUCTION
1. TEXTBOOK ANALYSIS
2. CLASSROOM ANALYSIS
3. STUDENT ANALYSIS

1. INTERVIEWS
2. SITUATIONAL ANALYSIS

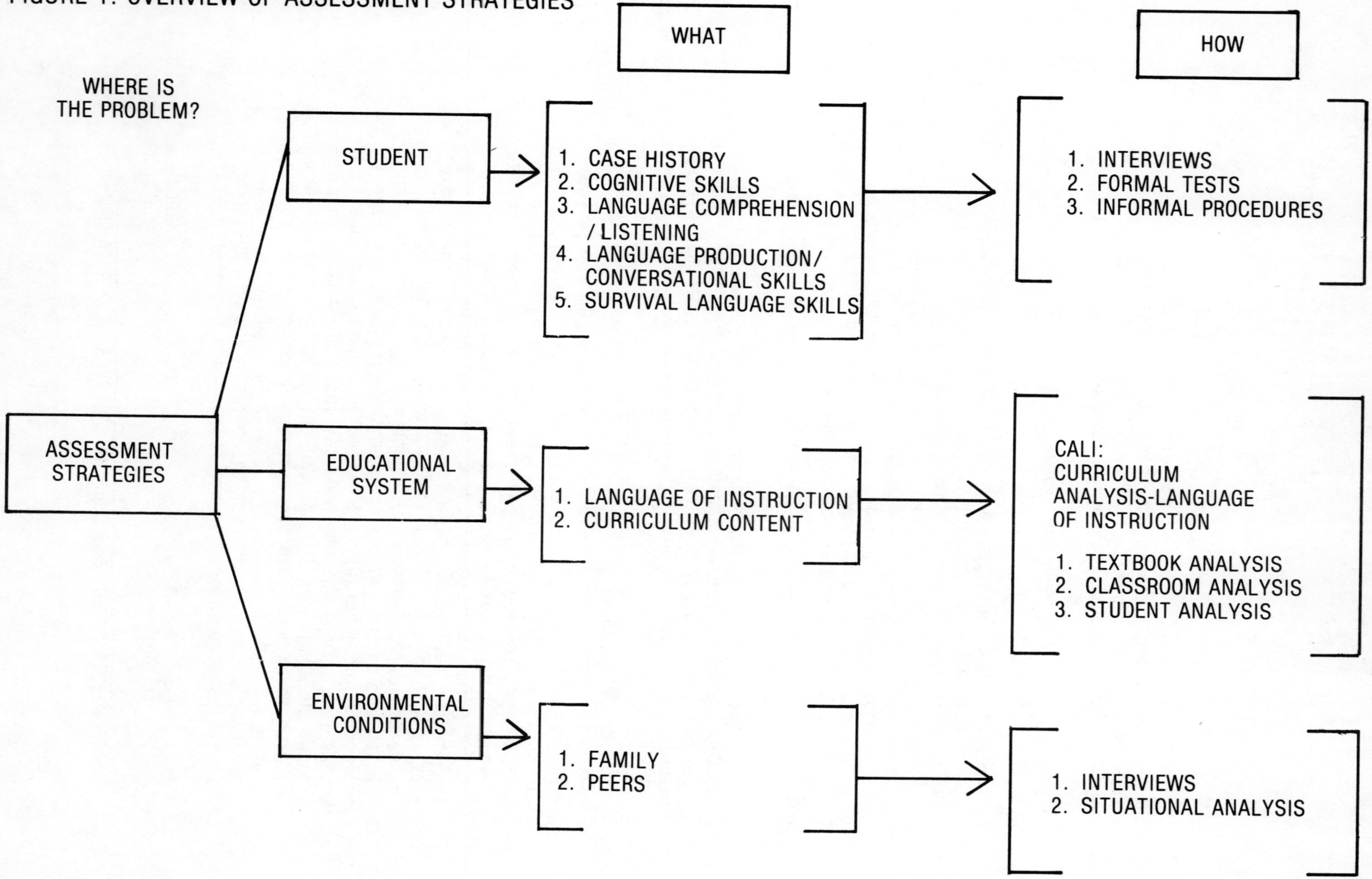

2. Our concept of typical adolescence is influenced by economic, legal, and sociocultural factors. Also, the period of time we live in influences our conception of "typical adolescence."

3. Adolescence is further influenced by the interaction between physiological, psychological, and environmental factors.

    a. Physiologically, this is the time in which the young person becomes sexually mature.

    b. Psychologically, adolescence is that period of time in which the person establishes independence from parental control and influence, and affiliates with the peer group. During this time, a personal identity, a value system, and an ideology develop providing preparation to cope with adulthood. Also, research has demonstrated that accelerated cognitive growth occurs during adolescence (Alley and Deshler, 1979).

    c. Environmental opportunities, demands, and stresses interact with individual characteristics to cause young people to act differently within the same sociological conditions.

4. It is imperative that educators working with the adolescent population understand this period of development.

C. Respond to the Adolescent's Individuality

Respond to the adolescent first as an individual rather than to the group of which he/she is a member.

D. Remember to Describe and Not Judge Behaviors

Remember to describe, not judge the adolescent's dress, posture, hair style, etc. Whenever value judgments are made, they should be under "impressions" in a diagnostic report and not stated as facts.

E. Do Not Approach the Adolescent as if You, Too, Were a Teenager

Adolescents do not respect you more for abandoning your professional role to be a "swinging" teenager (Emerik and Hatten, 1979).

33

F. Consider the Student's Right to Know About the Assessment Process

Explain how the information will be used to assist him/
her. Specifically explain to the student what behaviors
are to be assessed, how they are to be assessed, and the
reason for the various tests. The adolescent should be
made an active part of the evaluation process and encouraged to challenge and question what is being done (Emerik
and Hatten, 1979).

G. Listen to the Student's Perspective of the Problem

Listening closely to the student is important since he/
she may have insights into the problem that no one else
may have. Also, if there is a discrepancy between your
examination results and the student's perspective of the
problem, educational in-servicing or counseling may be
warranted prior to intervention.

H. Consider Variables That May Invalidate Results

Consider what variables may influence the student's performance in a negative way and thus invalidate results.
For example, consider medication type and the frequency
of administration, strenuous activities that precede
assessment, emotional stability at the time of assessment, and the day of the week that the evaluation occurred.

I. Assess the Student in More Than One Educational Setting

Consider the student's performance not only in the individual testing situation but also in the classroom, the
lunchroom, and the gymnasium. The adolescent's behavior
may change drastically depending upon the situation.

J. Assess the Student With A Variety of Familiar and Unfamiliar Listeners

Assess the student communicating with adults who are
familiar and unfamiliar and with peers who are familiar
and unfamiliar to the person.

K. Evaluate the Student's Communication Skills Across A
Variety of Communication Situations

1. Do not assess the language components of phonology
(sound system), morphology (free and bound morphemes),
syntax (word order), and semantics (meaning) as separate isolated behaviors such as many formal discrete
point tests do. A series of fragmented language
parts will not constitute the total communication
process.

34

2. Start with representative spontaneous language samples obtained from various communication situations. The whole can then be analyzed in terms of the various language components.

L. Realize When to Use Formal Standardized Tests, When to Use Informal Procedures, and When to Use Both

1. Standardized tests provide us with normative data which allows for calculation of scale scores or age equivalency. They provided a systematic procedure to compare a student to the peer group and determine the extent of the problem. Examiners should not consider administering standardized tests unless they can abide by the underlying theoretical assumptions. Standardized tests are not appropriate for all students due to:

   a. The rigidity of the methodology of the test

   b. Inappropriateness of population norms

2. Informal procedures allow for a great deal of flexibility in application. The testing procedures and materials can be modified to conform to the individual, rather than the individual conforming to the test procedures. However, informal procedures usually do not yield scaled scores.

3. The type of evaluation procedure you select depends upon the type of information you seek. For example, it may depend upon the availability of a particular assessment instrument.

4. One's educational training and personality may affect test selection. Training programs and supervisors tend to emphasize specific tests and procedures. Personal preference may also be a factor.

M. Make Praise Specific, Not General, in an Evaluation Session

Make praise contingent upon a particular evaluation task rather than making general statements such as, "You are a good worker." A specific statement would be, "I like the way you listened to my instructions."

N. Determine the Student's Optimum Learning Style

Is the student a better auditory, visual, tactile, or multi-sensory learner? Keep this optimum style in mind as assessment tasks are selected and completed.

O. Determine the Adolescent's Strengths as Well as Their
    Weaknesses

    It is a human need to be recognized for what we do well,
    not just for what we do wrong. Isolating strengths will
    often boost motivation and self-confidence on the part
    of the student. These strengths will be used to compen-
    sate for the weaknesses.

P. Establish A Comprehensive Multidisciplinary Team

    Appropriate professionals, the parents, and the student
    are members of the team.

Q. Discuss Results and Recommendations With the Student,
    the Parents, and Other Appropriate Professionals

    This discussion of the results of the evaluation and
    recommendations may be completed first with the student
    or together with the parents and school personnel. Do
    not exclude the student.

R. Consider the Adolescent's Frustrations With the Educa-
    tional System

    There is a real possibility that the adolescent is frus-
    trated and has a lowered self-esteem due to repeated aca-
    demic failure. This repeated academic failure may be a
    result of the educational system not recognizing the
    student's specific needs.

S. Recognize Decreased Parental Involvement But Increased
    Parental Concern

    It is not unusual to find a lessening of parental involve-
    ment with the adolescent but increased parental concern
    about academic achievement and vocational planning (Brown
    1978).

T. Recognize the Adolescent's Unwillingness to be Identified
    With A Special Group

    The adolescent may not appreciate being identified with a
    special group. Thus, remedial recommendations based upon
    the assessment results may be rejected.

IV. SUMMARY

An overview of the assessment process for adolescents reveals
that examiners need to first ask where the problem lies --
with the student, the educational system, and/or the environmental conditions. Assuming the problem is within the student
twenty general philosophical principles to apply with adolescents are presented. The principles stress the need for

36

adolescents to be active, informed participants in the assessment process. One might say there are no "hidden agendas" when it comes to assessing adolescents for language disorders.

V. ACTIVITIES

A. List any additional general philosophical principles under which you operate during the assessment process with adolescents.

1.

2.

3.

B. Analyze your current preferences with regard to use of formal tests versus informal procedures. Consider your population, agency requirements, clinical expertise, and personal needs.

	Formal Tests		Informal Tests
Pro:	1.	Pro:	1.
	2.		2.
	3.		3.
Con:	1.	Con:	1.
	2.		2.
	3.		3.

ASSESSMENT STRATEGIES: CASE HISTORY FORM

I. ## INTRODUCTION

Data needs to be accumulated on the student's past history, present status, and future goals. Only in this way can an accurate assessment protocol be planned for the student.

II. ## WHAT TO ASSESS

Information should be gathered in at least three key areas:

A. Medical data should be obtained on past and present medications, allergies, seizures, diseases, etc., that might affect performance.

B. An educational history should be collected on specific strengths and weaknesses in the academic subject areas. It should answer questions such as:

1. Did the person ever receive speech-language services? When? For how long?

2. What and how were oral language behaviors taught?

3. What was the student's reaction to such services?

4. Why was the person dismissed?

C. An environmental history should be accumulated on the family constellation, peer group status, and future vocational goals as they affect performance.

III. ## HOW TO ASSESS

Primarily, this information is obtained through written cumulative records and interviews with the student, parents, peers, special and general educators, medical personnel, social workers, and speech-language pathologists. Once this case history information has been obtained, it should be interpreted in light of the entire evaluation results. The following pages contain a sample case history form developed by the authors that is appropriate to use with adolescents.

IV. ## SUMMARY

The case history questions concern relevant information about adolescent students gathered from medical, educational, and environmental sources. Students themselves should provide as much of this information as possible.

CASE HISTORY FORM FOR ADOLESCENTS

Date:_____

I. Personal Information

A. Name: _____

B. Birthdate:_____ C. Age:_____ D. Sex:_____M _____F

E. Address: _____

F.   home:_____ work:_____

G. Education: Highest grade completed_____

H. List and describe below all members of your family.
Indicate in the far right column any speech, hearing, or language problems present among other members of the household.

Name	Relationship	Sex	Communication Problem

II. Educational History

A. Please list the school subjects you are the best in.

_____

B. Please list the school subjects you enjoy the most.

_____

C. Please list the school subjects you have the most difficulty in.

_____

D. Why do you feel you are having difficulty with these subjects?

_____

_____

E. Do you have any future vocational goals? _____No _____Yes
If yes, describe:_____

Larson, V. and Boyce, N. © 1983
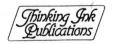

III. Health History

A. List below 1) major illnesses, diseases, or operations; 2) age at the time of each; and 3) resulting health complications or handicaps.

Illnesses/diseases/accidents	Age	Resulting handicaps
_____		_____
_____		_____
_____		_____

B. Were you hospitalized for any of the above conditions?
_____No _____Yes If so, where?_____
For how long?_____

C. Have you received, or are you now receiving rehabilitation treatment such as radiation therapy, physical therapy, occupational therapy? Describe the reason for, type, duration and result of treatments:_____

_____

_____

D. Are you currently under a doctor's care? _____No _____Yes

For what?_____

E. Are you currently taking any medication? _____No _____Yes

What kind?_____

For what?_____

How much?_____

How often?_____

40

F. Do you have any known allergies? _____No _____Yes

Describe:_____

G. Do you have any known drug sensitivities? _____No _____Yes

Describe:_____

H. Have you had seizures? _____No _____Yes How often?_____

When was the most recent seizure?_____

I. Do you have any known hearing problems? _____No _____Yes

Describe:_____

Hearing aid worn? _____No _____Yes

J. Do you have any known visual problems? _____No _____Yes

Describe:_____

Glasses worn? _____No _____Yes

IV. Present Speech, Language, or Hearing Problem

A. Describe the present problem.

B. How long has there been a problem?

C. What do you think caused the problem?

D. What types of speech and language services have you received?

How long have you received them?

E. Why were you dismissed from speech and language therapy?

F. How do you feel about your speech and language problem?

G. What is your primary means of communication?

H. Are you understood when you speak? If not, describe:

I. Do you understand when others talk to you? _____No _____Yes

    If not, describe:

J. Do you avoid speaking situations? _____No _____Yes

    Describe:

K. Are there times or situations when your problem is better or worse? _____No_____Yes

    Describe:

V. **Please provide in the space below any additional information which may be useful in evaluating your communication skills and in planning a therapy program.**

V. ACTIVITIES

    A. Based on your clinical observations, what additional information would be important to collect from the case history form?

        1.

        2.

        3.

    B. What agencies, clinics, services, programs, etc. have information that might be valuable regarding students you assess in your area?

        1.

        2.

        3.

        4.

        5.

        6.

    C. If you have not already established a working relationship with representatives from your list above, what strategies would you use to begin a cooperative exchange of information?

        1.

        2.

        3.

ASSESSMENT STRATEGIES: COGNITIVE SKILLS

I. INTRODUCTION

A. Rationale for Assessing and Teaching Cognition

Paging ahead to the sections on Assessment of Language Comprehension/Listening, Language Production/Conversational Skills, and Survival Language Skills would quickly reveal that specific cognitive skills are necessary prerequisites to many other oral communication behaviors. The authors believe there is a strong interplay between cognition and language. Therefore, a student's evaluation would be incomplete without assessment of cognitive skills. The idea of teaching cognition, or teaching someone to think, is viewed with skepticism by many educators. However, there is a growing body of research to support the benefits of teaching thinking skills to adolescents (Feuerstein, 1980; Lipman and Sharp, 1974; Ennis, 1965). A Stanford Research Institute report, Compensatory Education in Early Adolescence (1974), has shown that accelerated cognitive growth occurs during early adolescence and that students receiving intervention at that age may be receptive to ideas they previously did not grasp. Whether educators believe cognitive skills can be directly taught or not, most will agree that they can be enhanced by providing an environment in which they can develop.

B. Definition of Cognition/Cognitive Skills

Broadly defined, cognition is one's knowledge of the world and the mental processes of knowing and becoming aware of that world. Some prefer to define cognition in terms of potential for knowing and becoming aware (Feuerstein, 1980) rather than as a genetically predetermined factor.

C. Types of Cognition/Cognitive Skills

There are several types of cognitive skills (Feuerstein, 1980), each interrelated with the others:

1. Input, which involves collecting the information needed to solve a given problem.

2. Elaboration, which involves efficient utilization of that data.

3. Output, which involves communicating the solution or outcome of elaboration.

44

II. ADOLESCENTS AS THINKERS

   A. Early Adolescence

   Adolescents are in transition between concrete and formal operational periods of thought. Concrete thinkers have the following characteristics (Phillips, 1969; Gorman, 1972; Ginsburg and Opper, 1969):

     1. Decentration, or the ability to take another's perspective.

     2. Reversibility, or the ability to return a logical operation to its point of origin.

     3. Classification, or the ability to differentiate and coordinate essential properties of a set.

     4. Seriation, or the ability to sequence objects and events by a specific attribute.

     5. Causality, or the ability to understand cause-effect relationships.

     6. Conservation, or the realization that certain properties of a system remain the same in spite of transformations.

   B. Late Adolescence

   Formal thinkers have the following characteristics (Phillips, 1969; Gorman, 1972; Ginsburg and Opper, 1969):

     1. Hypothetical-deductive reasoning, or the ability to engage in "if-then" thinking and hypothesis generation.

     2. Second-order operations, or operating on operations (e.g., proportions, analogies).

     3. The 16 binary operations, or use of a combinatorial system, relating all possible solutions into a structured whole.

     4. INRC operations:

       a. Identity, or the realization that when applied to a function, it remains unchanged (e.g., $0 \times 3 = 0$).

       b. Negation, or the ability to draw a conclusion by thinking back to the original state (e.g., Friction causes moving objects to stop. If there is an absence of friction, there must be an absence of stopping.).

     c.   <u>Reciprocity</u>, or the realization that one factor can compensate for another (e.g., weight makes up for height, and vice versa).

     d.   <u>Correlativity</u>, or the interchange between conjunction (the combined presence of instances e.g., "both A and B") and disjunction (the choice of "either one or the other or both").

  5. <u>Meta-cognition</u>, or the ability to think about thinking.

C. <u>Transition</u>

Most adolescents begin making the transition from concrete to formal operational thought around 11 - 13 years of age although it may never be completed. Some studies have found about half of the adults in the United States either do not engage in formal operational thought, or do so only in their field of expertise (Lawson and Wollman, 1976; Labinowicz, 1980; Ritter, E., 1981).

D. <u>Sexual Differences</u>

On Piagetian tasks which require the application of formal operational thought, adolescent boys will consistently out-perform the girls (Elkind, 1975). Adolescent girls, perhaps for social role reasons, are more likely to apply their formal operational thinking to interpersonal matters than to matters of science. Elkind (1975) maintains that adolescents of average intellectual ability probably attain formal operations, but they do not apply them equally to all aspects of reality.

III. <u>WHAT TO ASSESS IN COGNITIVE SKILLS</u>

A. <u>Input</u>

It is suggested the following questions be asked with regard to the input skills of the adolescent (Feuerstein, 1980; Vermont, 1977; Vermont, 1979):

1. To what extent does the student fail to use clear perception (i.e., without seeming blurred and sweeping) to gather information?

2. To what extent does the student use unplanned, impulsive, or unsystematic behavior when gathering information?

3. To what extent does the student have impaired receptive verbal tools (i.e., lack of appropriate labels) for objects, events, and relationships?

4. To what extent does the student have impaired conservation of constancies (e.g., size, shape, orientation)?

5. To what extent does the student have impaired temporal, or time, concepts?

6. To what extent does the student have impaired spatial orientation?

7. To what extent does the student seem to lack precision and accuracy when gathering information?

8. To what extent does the student deal with data in a piecemeal fashion, failing to consider two or more sources of information at once?

9. To what extent does the student fail to gather and organize data on a given topic from a variety of sources?

B. Elaboration

It is suggested that the following questions be asked with regard to the elaboration skills of the adolescent (Feuerstein, 1980; Alley and Deshler, 1979):

1. To what extent does the student avoid using hypothetical-deductive reasoning (i.e., "if-then")?

2. To what extent is the student unaware when a problem exists and how to define the problem?

3. To what extent does the student lack the ability to analyze the problem and select relevant versus non-relevant cues?

4. To what extent does the student avoid developing options for solving the problem?

5. To what extent does the student lack spontaneous comparative behavior?

6. To what extent does the student seem to lack an ability to pursue logical evidence?

7. To what extent does the student appear to remain unchanged as a result of experiences encountered? For example, to what extent does the student solve a problem one day, but when faced with a similar problem the next day, find himself/herself unable to use the previously gathered information?

8. To what extent does the student seem to need concrete motor behavior when solving a problem?

9. To what extent does the student consider memory or remembering a "happening" that involves limited control by the individual? To what extent does the student describe his memory as either "there" or "not there?"

10. To what extent does the student seem to lack planning behavior?

11. To what extent does the student lack strategies for hypothesis testing?

12. To what extent does the student make inappropriate decisions based upon available information?

C. Output

It is suggested that the following questions be asked with regard to the output skills of the adolescent (Feuerstein, 1980; Alley and Deshler, 1979; Vermont, 1977; 1979):

1. To what extent does the student persist in using egocentric speech, failing to take the perspective of others?

2. To what extent does the student lack initiation of new responses or openly avoid encounters with stimuli that may lead to failure?

3. Upon making a decision, to what extent does the student execute the decision?

4. To what extent does the student use trial and error responses when a systematic approach would be more efficient?

5. To what extent does the student seem to lack precision and accuracy when communicating responses?

6. To what extent does the student have a deficiency in visual transport, the ability to complete a given figure by visually transporting a missing part from a distance or by choosing the missing part from a number of alternatives?

7. To what extent does the student appear to have difficulty summarizing the environment? For example, when asked "How many rooms are in your house?", the student will start to enumerate rooms rather than state the number.

8. To what extent does the student establish and grasp relationships in one situation, but fail to apply them in the handling of a new situation?

9. To what extent does the student lack the ability to summarize or draw conclusions from data provided on a chart, graph, table, map, or list of facts?

IV. HOW TO ASSESS COGNITIVE SKILLS

Input, elaboration, and output are interrelated, and it would be artificial to separate them for assessment purposes. Thus, this section will focus on the format used whether it be informal procedures or formal instruments. Within a suggested assessment task, all three types of skills (i.e., input, elaboration, and output) can be examined.

A. Informal Procedures

The following informal procedures are intended to comprise an appropriate, but not exhaustive, list of assessment activities to use with adolescents.

1. Gathering Data: Present the student with a multi-activity picture or diagram. Have the student describe what is seen. Have the student project what might be heard, smelled, or felt. Record responses. Note how precisely and accurately the student gathers the data.

2. Using Planned Behavior: Present a multi-sectioned picture or collage of individual photographs. Observe whether the student describes it in an organized systematic manner or exhibits unplanned, unsystematic behavior. Require that each picture be described. Look for the order used (e.g., "left to right," "top to bottom," "most appealing to least appealing").

3. Spatial Orientation: Have the student look at a map while you ask questions. Require "left-right" responses and "N-S-E-W" responses. A sample map and questions might be:

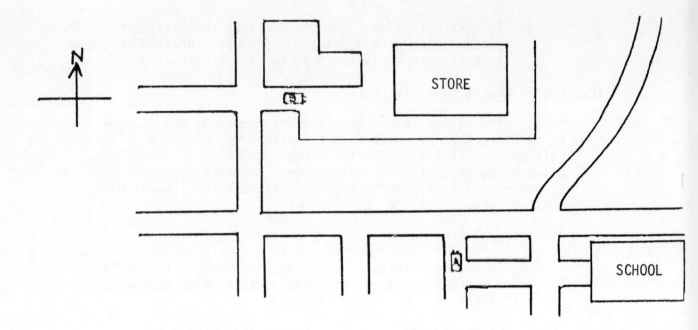

Example Questions:

In which direction is the car at the school (Car A) headed?

In which direction is the car at the store (Car B) headed?

What turns will Car A make to go to the store?

    4.   Problem Identification and Solution: Present situations that could occur and check for the student's ability to spontaneously use a problem solving model (Alley and Deshler, 1979).

        a. Identifying the problem

        b. Analyzing the problem

        c. Developing options for solving the problem

        d. Making a decision (choosing the best option)

        e. Executing the decision

Example situations might be:

Getting fired from a job and having a child to support.

Forgetting your billfold (and realizing it after you put gas in your car).

Having a project due for social studies tomorrow that you have not yet begun.

5. Comparisons/Categorization: Present the student with any two words and ask, "How are they alike?"; "How are they different?" (regardless of the word pair, an abstract thinker can make a comparison).

6. Organization:

    a. Given an assortment of words, have the student suggest one or more ways in which to organize the words (e.g., alphabetically, by linguistic categories, by function).

    b. Ask the student how a particular item(s) could be found in a grocery store, a department store, a shopping mall. Push for a variety of strategies.

    c. Ask the student, "Why do we organize?"; "What do we organize?"; "Can you think of anything we don't organize?"

7. Bridging: After you have discussed some cognitive functions such as taking the perspective of another person, or categorizing, ask, "Where else do you use that kind of thinking (in school) (outside of school)?" Observe whether the student can transfer the thinking skill to another situation.

8. Multiple Sources of Information: Present a table, a chart, or a graph with at least three variables. At first, ask the student specific questions that retrieve specific bits of data. Then ask the student to summarize all the information presented.

9. Inferential-Hypothetical Thinking: Engage the student in a "what if" discussion. Note the student's ability to engage in talking about a nonexistent, nonreal entity. (Examples: "What if the school burned down today?" "What if you had a child that was handicapped?" "What if your dad died?" "What if you were a whiz in mathematics?")

10. Piagetian Operations: Informal tasks are extensively described in Copeland (1974) and Wadsworth (1978). It is suggested that additional informal procedures be completed based on their recommended assessment tasks.

B. Formal Instruments

The following formal tests have been found to be appropriate for assessing cognitive ability in adolescents:

1. Instrumental Enrichment (Mastery Pages) and Dynamic Assessment of Retarded Performers (Feuerstein, 1980)

These instruments provide in-depth evaluation of all cognitive functions. Major drawbacks include the time it takes to administer them and the money required for training and materials costs.

2. Structure of Intelligence (SOI) (Meeker, 1975)

The SOI is an excellent tool for assessing cognitive skills. It includes a short screening test or a larger, in-depth test. Meeker has also made templates for a number of traditional intelligence tests. The templates isolate those items that are more indicative of potential for learning (i.e., what a child can learn versus what the child has already learned).

3. Detroit Tests of Learning Aptitude (Baker and Leland, 1967)

Selected subtests assess cognitive skills. Especially useful are pictorial and verbal absurdities, the orientation section, disarranged pictures, oral directions, and likenesses and differences.

4. Inventory of Essential Skills (Brigance, 1981)

This inventory is exhaustive in its approach to assessment of all major facets of daily living. Selected subtests reveal a considerable amount of information about a student's thinking skills in common situations (e.g., identifying and interpreting graphs, arranging numerals in numerical order, following bus schedules and map routes, converting recipes to different servings).

5. Psycho-Educational Battery - Part I (Woodcock and Johnson, 1977)

Part One "Tests of Cognitive Ability," provides a broad cognitive ability profile. Subtests that best address the questions asked in the "What to Assess" section are analysis-synthesis, concept formation, and analogies. The test has been normed on preschool through adult subjects.

6. Test of Concept Utilization (Crager, 1972)

The TCU provides qualitative and quantitative assessment of conceptual thinking by having students indicate similarities between pictures of common objects (e.g., a tree and an apple, a book and a horseshoe, a razor and a ticket). Standardized responses are provided as are norms for ages 5 - 18 years.

7. State Departments of Education

The Federal Government made reasoning/problem solving a basic skill in 1978. In response, a number of states are developing tests that students must pass in order to graduate from high school (e.g., Vermont, Utah). These tests can be additional sources for the field of communication disorders.

For example, the State of Utah (1978) has identified four life competency areas: consumer of goods and services, career, health and safety, and democratic governance. Within each of these areas, the basic skill area of problem solving has suggested performance indicators for measuring functional competency. For each of the problem solving tasks, the student presents orally, or in writing, a statement of the problem, other pertinent information, sources for further information, suggested action(s) to be taken, and a rationale for that action. From the health and safety competency area, one of the situations to which students are asked to respond involves finding a three-year-old child playing with a bottle of aspirin that was half full and is now empty with no aspirins found in the area.

V. SUMMARY

This section provides a rationale for assessing and teaching cognitive skills as well as data on what to assess and how to assess this behavior. The authors list available formal tests that might be used and present informal procedures for the reader's consideration.

VI. ACTIVITIES

A. What is happening in your state with regard to testing of reasoning/problem solving skills during grades 7-12?

1.

2.

3.

B. What kinds of thinking skills are deficient in your students (i.e. if you could change anything about the way your students presently think, what would it be)?

1.

2.

3.

C. Who do you consider to be a "good thinker" among the students you know?_____
What characteristics does that person(s) have that result in the label of "good thinker?"

1.

2.

3.

What characteristics do you consider indicative of a "poor thinker?"

1.

2.

3.

D. List additional informal procedures and formal instruments you have found useful when assessing cognitive skills in adolescents.

1.

2.

3.

ASSESSMENT STRATEGIES: LANGUAGE COMPREHENSION/LISTENING

I. INTRODUCTION

A. Rationale for Assessing and Teaching Listening

1. A review of the literature revealed that listening is the basic skill we engage in the highest percentage of the time; yet it is the least taught and most taken for granted of the basic skills of reading, writing, speaking, analyzing, and listening. According to Neville (1959) "more failure in academic and (personal) social growth can be traced to the inability to listen than to any other single aspect of the language arts." And yet, Oyer (1966) stated that listening is learned behavior and it can be concluded that it is a skill that can be taught.

2. It is important to consider listening in relation to:

a. Language Development

According to Lundsteen (1971), listening is the first language skill that we develop. As children, we listen before we speak, speak before we read, read before we write.

b. Time Spent On Listening

i. Wilt (1950) found elementary students are expected to listen 57.5% of the time in the classroom. Markgraf (1966) found that high school students are expected to spend 46% of their classroom time listening.

ii. Rankin (1926) found that adults spend 42.1% of their total verbal communication time listening, 31.9% speaking, 15% reading, and 11% writing.

iii. Werner (1975) conducted an update of the Rankin study. She found that 54.93% of the verbal communication time was spent listening, 23.19% speaking, 13.27% reading, and 8.40% writing.

c. Personal Development

   According to the Commission on English Curriculum of the National Council of Teachers of English, people's attitudes and concepts, whether they are economic, political, or ethical, are influenced and perhaps determined by their listening.

B. Definition of Listening

   1. It should be kept in mind that even though listening is itself a process, it is also an integral part of the total communication process.

   2. There have been many proposed definitions of listening. However, according to Wolvin and Coakley (1982) the definition of listening is still being developed. They feel that this current state of the art is due to the fact that "...listening is a complex, covert act difficult to investigate; much research in listening has not been coordinated or collated and research in listening is in an exploratory state -- with most of the research in listening having been conducted in the past four decades" (Wolvin and Coakley 1982, p. 30).

   3. A working definition of listening describes it as a process whereby a listener derives some type of meaning from the speaker's intent. The listener processes the message contingent upon his/her physiological, psychological, and sociological status; the situational context; and the type and degree of impinging noise.

C. Types of Listening

   The literature cites that there are several types of listening and that each type is not mutually exclusive of the other, but interrelated.

   1. Auditory perceptual

      a. Auditory attention

      b. Auditory figure-ground

      c. Auditory discrimination

      d. Auditory sequential memory

      e. Auditory synthesis

   2. Auditory comprehension of linguistic processes

56

3. Appreciative listening

4. Comprehensive/informational listening

5. Critical listening

6. Therapeutic listening

II. <u>ADOLESCENTS AS LISTENERS</u>

   A. <u>Characteristics That Facilitate Listening</u>

     1. Appropriate to most listening situations is the ability to:

       a. Hear and perceive sound

       b. Understand readily the meaning of words, sentences, and long units of oral expression

       c. Ask appropriate questions at appropriate times

       d. Be sensitive to the speaker's verbal and non-verbal behavior

       e. Concentrate attention on the material being presented in spite of lack of interest, fatigue, suspicion, or any physical, mental, or emotional problems

       f. Anticipate the sequence of ideas

       g. Associate ideas accurately

       h. Recall related experiences

       i. Recognize and interpret what may be called "oral punctuation"

       j. Give appropriate feedback to the speaker.

     2. Specific to the educational system, the student should:

       a. Initiate and continue developing the necessary vocabulary for the course content

       b. Adapt note taking or memory scheme to the individuality of the speaker's presentation

       c. Select the main points of the lecture

       d. Relate subordinate points to the main points of the lecture

e. Evaluate the content of the lecture critically and objectively

f. Retain the logical sequence of the topic and mentally maintain a running summary of the teacher's points

g. Ask mental questions and listen for their answers as the topic is discussed

B. Characteristics That Interfere With Listening

1. The student feels the subject is dull.

2. The student criticizes the speaker's looks, actions, and speaking style.

3. The student gets overstimulated or emotionally involved.

4. The student listens only for isolated facts.

5. The student tries to outline everything.

6. The student wastes the differential between speaking speed (150-200 words per minute) and thinking speed (400 words per minute).

7. The student listens only to what is easy to understand.

8. The student lets emotionally laden words get in the way.

9. The student becomes distracted.

10. The student permits personal prejudices to impair understanding.

III. WHAT TO ASSESS IN LISTENING SKILLS

The categories under A, B, and C in this outline were extrapolated from the work of Wiig and Semel (1976).

A. Auditory Acuity

1. To what extent is hearing affected at low and high frequencies?

2. To what extent is hearing affected at the speech frequencies?

B. Auditory Perception

1. Auditory Attention

a. To what extent does the student sustain auditory
    attention over reasonable periods of time and
    situations?

b. To what extent is the student's auditory atten-
    tion easily distracted by other stimuli?

2. Auditory Figure-Ground

a. To what extent does the presence of a competing
    background noise affect the student's perfor-
    mance on a listening task?

b. To what extent do various types of competing
    noises affect the student's ability to understand
    the speaker?

3. Auditory Discrimination

a. To what extent can the student discriminate dif-
    ferences in the frequency (pitch), intensity
    (loudness), rhythm, duration, and timbre (the
    quality given to a sound by its overtones)?

b. To what extent can the student discriminate spe-
    cific phonemes in words differing by one speech
    sound, such as cat and sat?

c. To what extent can the student identify conso-
    nants, vowels, and blends in the initial, final,
    or medial positions of words?

d. To what extent can the student discriminate be-
    tween initial consonants, final consonants,
    medial consonants, vowels, and/or consonant
    blends?

e. To what extent can the student discriminate the
    initial and final syllables of multi-syllabic
    words?

f. To what extent can the student identify and dis-
    criminate the number of syllables in words of
    increasing length?

4. Auditory Sequential Memory

    a. To what extent can the student retain sequence
        in a series of auditory stimuli consisting of
        digits, phonemes, words (related and unrelated),
        phrases, and syntactic structures and sentences?

    b. To what extent can the student recall and repeat
        series of auditory stimuli?

    c. To what extent can the student follow a series
        of oral directions of increasing length or com-
        plexity?

5. Auditory Synthesis

    a. To what extent can the student form words out of
        separated, articulated phonemes?

    b. To what extent can the student predict and for-
        mulate words where phonemes or syllables are
        missing?

    c. To what extent can the student predict, formu-
        late, and/or complete sentences when a word or
        words are missing?

C. Auditory Comprehension of Linguistic Processing

    1. Phonology

        See auditory discrimination items b, c, d; auditory
        sequential memory items a and b; auditory synthesis
        items a and b.

    2. Morphology

        a. To what extent can the student identify and dif-
            ferentiate morphological structure?

        b. To what extent can the student identify the
            separate words that are parts of compound words?

        c. To what extent can the student identify and dis-
            criminate among meaningful prefixes and suffixes
            in complex words?

        d. To what extent can the student discriminate among
            and identify inflectional suffixes (comparative -
            er; superlative - est; past tense - d, t, ed,
            etc.)?

E. To what extent can the student identify deriva-
tional suffixes (noun derivation - er, or, tion,
ion; adverb derivation - ly, y, etc.)?

3. Syntax

    a. To what extent can the student differentiate
grammatical phrases, clauses, and sentences from
those that are grammatically incorrect or incomplete?

    b. To what extent can the student discriminate among
the various sentence transformations (active,
declarative, interrogative, passive declarative,
negative, etc.)?

4. Semantics

    a. To what extent can the student comprehend selected
vocabulary items (parts of speech) such as verbs,
adjectives, prepositions, pronouns, etc.?

    b. To what extent can the student comprehend voca-
bulary items such as shades of meaning and multiple-
meaning words, antonyms, synonyms, and homonyms?

    c. To what extent can the student comprehend linguis-
tic concepts requiring logical operations such as
comparative sentences, if-then constructions, etc?

    d. To what extent can the student process and compre-
hend verbal analogies expressing logical relationships between words and concepts?

    e. To what extent can the student process and compre-
hend sentences that express logical relationships
(comparative, passive, spatial, temporal, or famil-
ial) between words or elements?

    f. To what extent can the student process and compre-
hend sentences containing linguistic concepts of
inclusion-exclusion (some, none, all, any, all
except, etc.) or concepts such as if/then, either/
or, because, or when/then?

    g. To what extent can the student understand idioms,
metaphors, similes, and/or proverbs?

D. Comprehensive (Informational) Listening

1. To what extent does the student want to listen to
factual information?

61

2. To what extent is the student ready to concentrate his/her attention on the speaker?

3. To what extent does the student put the time difference between thinking and speaking speed to work to his/her advantage?

4. To what extent does the student listen primarily for global ideas rather than details?

5. To what extent does the student have the ability to pick out the main idea in a paragraph?

6. To what extent does the student understand how to relate details, examples, and illustrations to the global ideas?

7. To what extent does the student demonstrate the ability to allow the speaker to develop an idea before reacting to it?

8. To what extent does the student demonstrate the ability to adapt his/her note taking to the speaker?

9. To what extent does the student have an adequate listening vocabulary and the ability to remember and write factual information in each of the following concept areas: numbers and numeral relationships; letters, sounds, abbreviations, spelling and alphabetizing; directions and spatial relations; time and temporal sequence, dates and chronological order; measurements and amounts; proportion, comparison and contrast (Morley, 1975)?

E. Critical (Evaluative) Listening

1. To what extent is the student aware of external characteristics of the speaker that may be misleading (e.g., status of the speaker, personality, appearance)?

2. To what extent is the student aware of how perceived attitudes and prejudices toward the subject distort the message?

3. To what extent is the student aware of how multiple meanings of words affect interpretation of the speaker's message?

4. To what extent is the student a good critical listener as described in the list below?

a. The student can detect false reasoning (i.e. discriminate between fact and opinion; recognize false or weak analogies; detect hasty generalization; recognize either/or thinking; recognize cause and effect; recognize equivocation; detect wishful thinking; recognize rationalization).

b. The student can recognize and use inductive and deductive reasoning (i.e., recognize inductive reasoning: particular to general; recognize deductive reasoning: general to specific).

c. The student can recognize propaganda devices (i.e., be aware that listeners are more vulnerable than readers; recognize loaded words, name calling, slogans, "bandwagon" techniques, "plain folks," card stacking, transfer, testimonial speech).

F. Appreciative Listening

This is not an area to be assessed by speech-language pathologists, but added here for information. Wolvin and Coakley (1982) define appreciative listening as a highly individualized process of listening in order to obtain sensory stimulation or enjoyment through the works and experiences of others. What is appreciative listening for one person is not for another. Essentially, appreciative listening can include listening to music, the oral style of a speaker, environmental sounds, oral interpretation of literature, theater or radio, television and film.

G. Therapeutic Listening

This is added not for purposes of assessing the student, but rather for the speech-language pathologist to evaluate his/her own ability as an empathic listener. Some of the skills involved in therapeutic listening are: avoiding evaluative feedback; becoming an active listener; listening empathetically and non-directively; developing a supportive communication climate; paraphrasing messages and listening for feelings (Wolvin and Coakley, 1982).

IV. HOW TO ASSESS LISTENING SKILLS

A. Auditory Acuity

An audiologist may assess the following via appropriate instrumentation: pure-tone thresholds, sound localization, speech-reception thresholds, and speech discrimination.

B. <u>Auditory Perception</u>

   1. Formal Procedures

      a. <u>Detroit Tests of Learning Aptitude</u> (Baker and Leland, 1967)

         Auditory Attention Span for Unrelated Words Subtest; Oral Commissions Subtest; Auditory Attention Span for Related Syllables; Oral Directions.

      b. <u>Examining for Aphasia</u> (Eisenson, 1954)

         Subtest on Recognition of Sounds

      c. <u>Durrell Analysis of Reading Difficulty</u> (Durrell, 1955)

         Subtest on Hearing Sounds in Words

      d. <u>Gates-McKillop Reading Diagnostic Test</u> (Gates and McKillop, 1962)

         Subtest of: Syllabication

      e. <u>Revised Token Test</u> (McNeil and Prescott, 1978)

   2. Informal Procedures

      The examiner should observe and record behaviors across a series of educational situations and answer each item regarding what to assess in auditory perceptual skills.

C. <u>Auditory Comprehension of Linguistic Processing Skills</u>

   1. Formal Procedures

      a. Phonology (see the formal tests listed under Auditory Perception)

      b. Morphology-Syntax

         i. <u>Grammatical Comprehension Test</u> (Miller and Yoder, 1973)

        ii. <u>Revised Token Test</u> (McNeil and Prescott, 1978)

       iii. <u>Language Assessment Tasks</u> (Kellman, Flood and Yoder, 1978)

iv. Clinical Evaluation of Language Functions
(Semel and Wiig, 1980)

Processing Word and Sentence Structure

c. Cognitive-Semantic

  i. Peabody Picture Vocabulary Test - Revised
  (Dunn, 1980)

  ii. Botel Reading Inventory
  (Botel, 1970)

  Word opposites: Reading - Listening Subtest

  iii. Detroit Tests of Learning Aptitude
  (Baker and Leland, 1967)

  Subtests of: Verbal Absurdities; Verbal
  Opposites; Auditory Attention Span for
  Unrelated Words; Oral Commissions; Social
  Adjustment A and B; Orientation, Auditory
  Attention Span for Related Syllables; Oral
  Directions and Likenesses and Differences

  iv. Psycho-Educational Battery Parts I & II
  (Woodcock and Johnson, 1977)

  Subtests of: Memory for Sentences; Blend-
  ing; Antonyms; Synonyms; Numbers Reversed;
  Analogies; Science; Social Studies; Humani-
  ties

  v. Language Assessment Tasks
  (Kellman, Flood and Yoder, 1978)

  Subtests of: Language Comprehension of Syntax; Semantics; Paralinguistics and Language
  Content; and Auditory Memory

  vi. Clinical Evaluation of Language Functions
  (Semel and Wiig, 1980)

  Subtests of: Processing Word and Sentence
  Structure; Processing Word Classes; Processing Linguistic Concepts; Processing Relationships and Ambiguities; Processing Oral Directions; Processing Spoken Paragraphs; Producing Model Sentences; Processing Speech Sounds

       vii.   Test of Adolescent Language
               Hammill, Brown, Larsen, and Wiederholt, 1980)

               Subtest of: Listening/Vocabulary; Listening/Grammar

      viii. Inventory of Essential Skills
               (Brigance, 1981)

               Subtest of: Oral Communication and Telephone Skills

  2. Informal Procedures

    a. The examiner should use either object manipulation tasks or picture-pointing response modes to assess the student's ability to understand these structures: commands of increasing complexity and syntactical types; multiple meaning words; idiomatic expressions; conjunctives in sentences (and, or, but, if-then).

    b. The examiner should observe and record behaviors across a series of conversational/educational situations and answer each item regarding what to assess in auditory comprehension of linguistic processing skills.

D. Informational Listening

  1. Formal Procedures

    a. Brown-Carlsen Listening Comprehension Test
       (Brown and Carlsen, 1955)

    b. Sequential Tests of Educational Progress
       (Educational Testing Service, 1958)

    c. School Council Oracy Project
       (Wilkinson, Stratta, and Dudley, 1974)

  2. Informal Procedures

    a. The examiner should determine if the student can remember the main idea of a story and any details, examples, etc., supportive of the main idea.

    b. The examiner should determine if the student can remember factual concepts of number, time, space, etc. in a paragraph or story.

    c. The examiner should observe and record behaviors across a series of conversational/educational situations and answer each item regarding what to assess in auditory perceptual skills.

66

E. Critical Listening

1. Formal Procedures

    Presently, we have no formal tests devised to assess
    the critical listening area in junior/senior high
    school students except pre- and post-tests within
    listening programs. However, these tests do not spe-
    cifically assess each area, nor are they normed to
    meet the needs of professionals serving the handi-
    capped.

2. Informal Procedures

    a. The student could present and analyze speeches
        using various types of false reasoning and pro-
        paganda devices.

    b. The examiner should observe and record behaviors
        across a series of conversational/educational
        situations and answer items regarding what to
        assess in critical listening skills.

V. CRITIQUE OF COMMERCIAL TESTS

A. What stimulus items are used to elicit a listening re-
    sponse?

B. What response modes are used to determine if listening
    has occurred?

C. Is there normative data available on the types of stu-
    dents you are assessing?

D. What is the pragmatic value of this test?

VI. CRITERIA FOR ESTABLISHING AN "IDEAL" LISTENING TEST

A. Critical characteristics include: validity; reliability;
    standardization procedures; communication pragmatics;
    and the congruency of the theoretical constructs in rela-
    tion to the examiner's beliefs.

B. Desirable characteristics include: clear and concise
    instruction; ease in administering and scoring; economy
    in terms of student time and energy; availability of
    needed materials; and avoidance of cultural and sexual
    stereotyping.

VII. <u>SUMMARY</u>

This section provides a rationale for assessing and teaching
language comprehension/listening skills as well as data on
what to assess and how to assess this behavior. The authors
list available formal tests that might be used, and present
informal procedures for the reader's consideration.

VIII. ACTIVITIES

A. What is happening in your state with regard to testing of language comprehension/listening skills during grades 7 - 12?

   1.

   2.

   3.

B. What kinds of listening skills are deficit in your students (i.e., if you could change anything about the way your students presently listen, what would it be)?

   1.

   2.

   3.

C. Who do you consider to be a "good listener" among the students you know?_____

   What characteristics does that person(s) have that results in the label of "good listener?"

   1.

   2.

   What characteristics do you consider indicative of a "poor listener?"

   1.

   2.

D. List additional informal procedures and formal instruments you have found useful when assessing language comprehension/listening skills in adolescents?

   1.

   2.

   3.

ASSESSMENT STRATEGIES: LANGUAGE PRODUCTION/CONVERSATIONAL SKILLS

I. INTRODUCTION

A. Rationale for Assessing and Teaching Language Production/ Conversational Skills

The average person spends approximately 23% of the day engaged in speaking (Werner, 1975). While some of this speaking may involve delivering information verbally (e.g., speeches, lectures, presentations), for most people the bulk of the 23% is time spent in conversation. Despite the traditional importance of reading, writing, and mathematics, in a society moving at an increasing rate toward sound and pictures as primary modes of input, direct attention to spoken skills is of prime value. For survival in the world beyond school, one needs to have an adequate method whereby ideas, opinions, and feelings can be expressed in a socially acceptable manner. The most efficient system is the use of effective verbal communication. If you think for a minute, there are thousands of ways of earning a living, and effective speech is essential to every one.

B. Definition of Language Production/Conversational Skills

For purposes of this manual, the authors are defining language production as the morphological, syntactical, and semantic rules that one uses during oral expression. Certainly production of the language also involves phonology, as well as voice and fluency characteristics, but these areas are not addressed in more than a superficial way within the confines of this publication. Similarly, language production of adolescents from various etiological populations is not considered as a separate issue.

Conversational skills are being defined as the ability to function effectively as both speaker and listener when interacting orally with another person, using all the appropriate rules for conversation (Grice, 1975). They include saying the right words at the right time in the right way, as well as responding appropriately as a listener (see Assessment Strategies: Language Comprehension/ Listening section). A successful conversation will result in communication, the meeting of meaning between two or more people.

C. Functions of Language Production/Conversational Skills

An effective way to globally assess language production/
conversational skills is to consider whether students use
their verbal expression to convey each of the functions
of language using appropriate linguistic features in an
acceptable manner.

1. The functions of communication according to Hymes
   (1971) are listed below:

   a. To give information

   b. To get information (i.e., question asking)

   c. To describe an ongoing event

   d. To get one's listener to do, believe, or feel
      something (i.e., persuasion)

   e. To express one's own intentions, beliefs, and
      feelings (i.e., self-disclosure)

   f. To indicate a readiness for further communication

   g. To solve problems

   h. To entertain

2. Searle (1976) discussed five major categories of speech
   acts:

   a. Representatives, statements that can be catego-
      rized as true or false

   b. Directives, statements in which the speaker attempts
      to get the listener to do something

   c. Commissives, statements that commit the speaker
      to some future action

   d. Expressives, statements that express psychologi-
      cal states

   e. Declarations, statements in which saying makes
      it so

3. In addition to the functions of speech, there are two
   conventions that govern speech acts among middle class
   standard American English speakers:

a. An obligation to be clear and informative

b. An obligation to be polite

II. ADOLESCENTS AS LANGUAGE PRODUCERS/CONVERSATIONALISTS

Before we can determine the existence of a language disorder,
we need to determine the language standard or norm to which
it is being compared.

A. Characteristics of Normal Adolescents

1. Larson and Boyce (in preparation) analyzed conversational speech produced by normal 13-year old students
when they talked with each other and when they talked
with an unfamiliar adult of the opposite sex. The
following observations were made:

a. When talking with a friend of their choice, the
language functions "to give information," "to
get information," and "to describe one's beliefs,"
were used most frequently by all subjects. When
talking with an unfamiliar adult, the language
functions "to give information," and "to describe
one's beliefs," were used more frequently by all
subjects.

There was a marked lack of the function "to get
information" when the subjects spoke with an unfamiliar adult. All subjects were found to use
the function "to entertain" with peers, but rarely
with adults.

b. All subjects asked a significantly higher number
of questions when talking with their friends than
with an unfamiliar adult.

c. All subjects used a higher frequency of figurative language including idioms, slang, and humor
with their friends than they did with the unfamiliar adult.

d. All subjects used roughly equivalent time speaking in simple sentences, complex sentences, and
fragments. Run-on sentences containing a high
frequency of words such as "and" and "and so"
were common.

e. Verbal mazes were used with approximately equal
frequency within all conversations.

72

f. All subjects were considerably more likely to shift conversational topics with their peers than they were with the unfamiliar adults. At least half of the topic shifts completed between peers were of an abrupt nature, having no transition sentence to cue the listener that a new topic was about to begin.

g. Nonspecific language occurred with higher frequency between students and unfamiliar adults and with lesser frequency between peers. This may indicate some failure on the part of the subjects to consider the communication needs of the adult listeners.

2. MacWhinney and Bates (1978) have identified these devices for signaling old and new information used by those who are approximately 8 years old and older:

a. Ellipsis -- information may be indexed by deleting or omitting linguistic material as in this example:

   "Where are my car keys?"

   "In the ignition."

b. Pronominalization -- upon hearing pronouns, the listener is required to identify the specific referent from the context of previous linguistic material.

c. Emphatic Stress -- new information may be marked in spoken sentences by stressing specific items. Stress is frequently used where new information contrasts with earlier information. For example:

   "Instead of wine, let's order some champagne."

d. Indefinite Articles -- that a noun represents new information may be signaled by the use of an indefinite article. For example:

   "Charles bought a new car."

e. Definite Articles -- when a noun conveys given or old information, the definite article so indicates. For example:

   "The car is parked in the driveway."

73

f. <u>Initialization</u> -- where the language offers alternatives, adults seem to prefer placing known information before new information given in previous sentences. For example:

"That boy you saw is my son."

3. Rees and Wollner (1982) identified a taxonomy of conversational abilities that would already be part of a normal adolescent's repertoire:

a. To follow the conventions of sequential organization in conversation.

    i. Participating in conversation or interaction

    ii. Observing the rules of turn taking

    iii. Using conventional and effective means to open conversations

    iv. Responding to others' opening conversational moves

    v. Ending conversational sequences to bring conversations to a close

b. To engage in coherent conversation

    i. Distinguishing between old and new information

    ii. Establishing a topic for conversational exchange

    iii. Maintaining the topic across speaker utterances

    iv. Making relevant conversational contributions

c. To repair conversational errors

    i. As speaker, repairing unsuccessful conversational contributions

    ii. As listener, providing feedback about unsuccessful conversational contributions

d. To establish and vary role in relation to listener

    i. Using devices that express politeness or the lack of it

      ii.   Expressing meaning indirectly

     iii.   Switching codes as needed

  e. To produce and comprehend speech acts

       i.   Controlling a full range of elocutions

      ii.   Observing rules of appropriateness

     iii.   Conveying referential information effectively

4. Rees and Wollner (1982) also identified the rules of turn taking in conversation which should be well established by adolescence:

  a. Speaker exchange occurs and reoccurs. If there are two participants, both must have turns at speaking; if the participants number more than two, it is not required that all take turns at speaking.

  b. For the most part, only one speaker speaks at a time. If two or more speakers start simultaneously all but one drop out.

  c. The participant who is not speaking pays attention to the one who is speaking. Paying attention may take the form of:

       i.   Turning toward the speaker

      ii.   Looking at the speaker

     iii.   Not interrupting

      iv.   Acknowledging understanding by nonverbal cues (e.g., nodding, appropriate change of facial expression) or verbal cues (e.g., repetition or saying, "uh-huh")

       v.   Performing an action related to the speaker's content

  d. Gaps between speakers' turns are brief or nonexistent.

  e. Transitions from speaker to speaker are orderly.

  f. If overlap interferes with understanding, repair takes place. The overlap material may be spoken more slowly or more loudly, or may be repeated. To avoid interfering with comprehension during over-

lapping turn beginnings, the speaker frequently employs such starters as "well,"
"you know," "let me say that."

5. Chappell (1980) examined oral language performance
    obtained from a story reformulation task. His sub-
    jects spanned from fourth to seventh grade. Students
    who performed within normal limits for their grade
    level demonstrated:

    a. Appropriate pragmatic cognizance of what had to be
        retold (semantic aspects/interrelationships)

    b. Understanding of how it had to be said (skillful
        use of mature syntactic structures)

6. Loban (1976) completed a longitudinal study of 211 stu-
    dents that he tracked from Kindergarten through Grade 12.
    His major findings are as follows:

    a. Using communication units as his basic measurement,
        each year he charted the average number of words
        per unit. He found that a year of growth was typi-
        cally followed by a plateau, then by another year
        of growth.

    b. In analyzing the verbal mazes that his subjects
        used, he found that students ended Grade 12 with
        virtually identical percentages of verbal mazes
        that they had used in Grade 1. He found erratic
        upward and downward fluctuations during the middle
        years of school (Grade 4-9 or 10).

    c. Those students who were superior in oral language
        skills in Kindergarten and Grade 1 before they
        learned to read and write were the same students
        who excelled in reading and writing by the time
        they were in Grade 6.

    d. Loban supported the idea of stages of language
        development in such matters as continued growth in
        the average number of words per communication unit,
        the average of units, and the average number of
        dependent clauses. He found a steady growth during
        the elementary years followed by a plateau in Grades
        7-10, and a renewal or even greater growth velocity
        in Grades 11-12.

    e. He identified the adjective clause as the mark of
        increasing language development, both oral and
        written.

f. He found that regression in language can and will occur such as in situations of social threat.

g. When teachers were asked to describe "High" language users, they included these characteristics:

   i.   Remained in control of ideas expressed

   ii. Used a variety of vocabulary

   iii. Adjusted pace to listeners' needs

   iv. Spoke freely, fluently, effectively

   v.   Had a plan for their talking

   vi. Were attentive listeners

h. When teachers were asked to describe "Low" language users, they included these characteristics:

   i.   Rambled without apparent purpose

   ii. Seemed unaware of listeners' needs

   iii. Used meager vocabulary

   iv. Projected a hesitant, faltering style

7. Wiig (1982) has identifed these characteristics of adolescents in her studies:

   a. By 13 years, there is communicative maturity. A switch can be made between peer register and adult register and between formal and informal register.

   b. By 15 years, students use formal register for both peers and adults unless peers are their closest friends.

8. McCroskey (1981) analyzed normative levels of communication apprehension for students in Grades K-12. The study found that students in Kindergarten to Grade 3 feel significantly less fear communicating in school classrooms than do those in Grades 4-12. Some factor or combination of factors help increase communication apprehension during the early elementary school years that continues into adulthood. McCroskey indicated that the factors may involve peer contact and teacher behavior. The same study analyzed educators and found a significantly larger proportion of teachers in Grades K-4 with high communication apprehension than there

were teachers in these grades with low communication apprehension. A significantly larger proportion of high apprehensive teachers were in Grades K-4 than in either Grades 5-9 or Grades 10-12.

9. Willis and Garrison (1970) compared a group of normal adolescents with a group labeled "educable mentally retarded." They found the normal students used longer sentences and a greater variety of words. They also had fewer grammatical errors, but not at a significant level. Normal subjects had a mean sentence length of 12.59 words and a grammatical correction ratio of .98.

10. Johnson, et al. (1980) studied students at Grades 3, 6, and 9 and found the following:

    a. Recognition that an act of communication may be offensive appears to develop before the understanding of how to make such communication inoffensive. The ability to recognize an inept communication act appears to be well established by the third grade. At the sixth grade level, the ability to improve inept communication catches up with the ability to recognize ineptness.

    b. It was more difficult for subjects to correct inept attempts to make others feel better than it was to correct inept attempts to influence others' actions (e.g., It wasn't until ninth grade that students were able to correct more difficult inept stories such as: "Tom is sad because his dog died. You say, 'Cheer up, it's nothing to be upset about. Pretty soon you'll forget all about it.' " Students in sixth grade were able to handle easier stories such as: "You're studying for a test at school. Lou calls you up and wants to come over to visit. You say, 'You picked a fine time to visit.' ").

11. Dorval (1980) analyzed the conversational qualities of students spanning from second grade through late college. Conversational turns were categorized as unrelated and tangential, related, factual evaluation/elaboration/ question, perspective-oriented evaluation/elaboration/ question. The following results were found:

    a. Unrelated and tangential remarks occurred with appreciable frequency only at the youngest grade level studied, second grade.

    b. Related remarks increased in frequency during the elementary school years, then decreased in frequency as more complex topic-relations came to the fore in high school.

c. More complex remarks -- factual and perspective-
    oriented evaluations/elaborations/questions --
    first reached a sizable proportion during conver-
    sational speech in Grade 9, and increased steadily
    in frequency thereafter. Ninth graders' conversa-
    tion had a high proportion of evaluation comments
    relative to elaboration; that proportion declined
    thereafter.

d. Evaluations, elaborations, and questions that
    focused on people's perspectives or feelings were
    less frequent than those that focused on factual
    matters. They appeared with noticeable frequency
    only in late high school and adulthood.

12. French (1978) has been studying nonverbal patterns in
    the youth culture. He contends that the nonverbal
    patterns of normal adolescents today are quite differ-
    ent from those in the past. He indicates these non-
    verbal behaviors as being normal in today's adolescents:

a. The Black Walk: French maintains that many normal
    adolescents have developed a Black Walk probably as
    a result of the changing cultural patterns bringing
    Black Americans to the forefront in our country.
    He defines this walk as much slower than the White
    Walk -- actually, more of a stroll. The walker's
    head is often slightly elevated and tipped to one
    side, casually. Weight is cast to the heel of the
    rear foot. One arm swings with the hand slightly
    cupped. The other arm and hand hang limply or the
    hand is tucked in a pocket with the thumb outside.
    The gait is almost a walking dance.

b. The Blank Stare: The eyes of the student are focused
    beyond the listener when engaging in a conversation.

c. Back Turn: There is a shift in body position to
    slightly expose one's back to the receiver while
    engaging in conversation. In Black interactions,
    the back turn has been a sign of trust and has been
    used to signify understanding of what has been said.

d. The Eye Roll: Once used as an expression of dis-
    approval or impudence, the eye roll is used so exten-
    sively now by some adolescents that the message it
    once conveyed may be weakened.

French encourages educators to understand nonverbal
patterns in today's youth culture and to stay abreast
with what is common to the mainstream.

B. Minimal Speaking Skills

An increasing number of states and communities are establishing sets of nominal expectations of adolescents completing high school including requirements in the area of speaking. These minimal speaking skills can provide a helpful guide for identifying what is expected of normal adolescents. Those secondary level students who show a vast discrepancy between where they are now versus where they are expected to be at age 18 may be target students for identification and assessment. Examples of skills expected in several states are outlined below:

1. Vermont List (1977)

    a. Given a choice of familiar geographical locations, the student will give clear and accurate directions for reaching the selected location.

    b. Given directions to explain a process, make a report, or express an opinion, the student will do so, demonstrating organization, sequence, clarity, and accuracy.

    c. Given a simulated situation, the student will demonstrate the ability to answer a business telephone correctly and to take a message.

    d. Given a simulated situation, the student will demonstrate the ability to get information or assistance by using a telephone.

    e. Given a simulated situation, the student will demonstrate the ability to introduce himself/herself and others.

    f. Given a job interview situation, the student will respond to questions about his/her qualifications, experiences, and interests and will ask relevant questions.

    g. Given an informal discussion situation, the student will participate, listening to others, making suitable responses, and speaking loudly and clearly enough to be heard by all with whom he/she is communicating.

2. Minnesota List (1982)

    The student should apply oral communication skills in a variety of settings for several purposes:

a. The student should recognize that two-person interaction is the basis of all communication.

b. The student should understand the effective use of the voice.

c. The student should understand communication acts which cast participants in imaginary situations.

d. The student should understand communication acts in which the participants offer or seek information.

e. The student should understand the communication acts which express and respond to feelings and attitudes.

f. The student should understand the communication acts which serve to maintain social relationships and to facilitate social interaction.

g. The student should understand the communication acts which control behavior.

3. Oral Proficiency Program - Gary Community School Corporation (1977)

a. Students will be able to speak clearly and fluently.

b. Students will be able to avoid gross mispronunciation of common words. (Example: He axed me to go. We will git the groceries.).

c. Students will be able to talk without using non-meaningful verbal crutches. (Example: you know, like, like that, and --uh.)

d. Students will be able to talk at a rate that can be understood.

e. Students will be able to use words according to standard usage. (Examples of nonstandard usage: He seen the accident. I done my work.)

f. Students will be able to speak in a pleasant and natural voice.

g. Students will be able to speak loudly enough to be heard.

h. Students will be able to speak in complete sentences.

C. Language Production as Specified by the School Curriculum

A growing number of states are isolating specific speaking skills to emphasize at each grade level. As with the minimal competency lists, the information outlined below will provide the reader with insight into what is expected of normal adolescents:

1. Some Essential Learner Outcomes in Communications/ Language Arts (Minnesota, 1982)

    a. Grades 5-8

        i. The student should be able to perform improvisations, create and perform a story, perform stories from other cultures, and role play an event from history.

        ii. The student should be able to summarize pertinent information, give concise and accurate directions, organize messages so others can understand them, choose and introduce an appropriate topic for an informative talk, and effectively conclude an informative talk.

        iii. The student should be able to describe his/ her own perceptions, use nonverbal signs appropriate for a situation, and describe differences in expressing feeling.

        iv. The student should be able to identify ritual communication as opposed to other types of communication, participate in culturally appropriate communication rituals, and lead a group discussion.

        v. The student should be able to use persuasive arguments, support a position with appropriate arguments, support arguments with appropriate evidence, and analyze an audience.

    b. Grades 9-12

        i. The student should be able to identify when speaking is a joint venture (two or more persons), intrapersonal (internal monologue), interpersonal (two or more person dialogue), or continuous feedback.

        ii. The student should be able to evaluate vocalizations with regard to pitch and quality.

iii. The student should be able to conduct a formal meeting.

iv. The student should practice small group processing and public speaking.

2. Communication Skills Chart (Arizona, 1980)

a. Grades 7-9

i. The student tells how language is used in various occupations.

ii. The student recognizes complete sentences.

iii. The student identifies singular and plural pronouns.

iv. The student identifies adjectives and adverbs.

v. The student identifies possessive pronouns.

vi. The student identifies prepositions and objects of prepositions.

vii. The student discusses his reading with others.

viii. The student gives oral reports.

b. Grades 10-12

i. The student describes skills required for a particular vocation.

ii. The student fills out forms (e.g., driver's license, job application, savings account).

iii. The student applies interviewing skills (e.g., job, credit application).

iv. The student can speak before a group.

3. Other states that have produced a sequence of skills for speaking/listening are the following. You may wish to send for their information by writing to these State Departments of Education:

a. Illinois

b. Massachusetts

c. Michigan

83

            d. Pennsylvania

            e. Texas

        4. What oral language curriculum has your state developed?
            List specific skills cited and grade levels below:

            a.

            b.

            c.

            d.

            e.

            f.

            g.

III. WHAT TO ASSESS IN LANGUAGE PRODUCTION/CONVERSATIONAL SKILLS

    A familiarity with what is normal and expected during adoles-
    cence makes it possible to better assess the student. Examiners
    will want to determine if the student falls far below language
    production expectations as specified by the academic curriculum
    or by cultural and societal expectations.

    A. Linguistics

        During assessment, the following questions can be asked
        about these features:

84

1. Sentences

   a. To what extent does the student use complete, fully grammatical sentences?

   b. When sentence fragments are used, to what extent are they appropriate (e.g., a single word response to a "what+be" question is appropriate)? To what extent does the fragment leave the listener wondering what the message is?

   c. To what extent does the student use complex sentences that include embedded clauses or does the student simply conjoin short, simple sentences together with "and," "and so," etc.?

2. Questions

   a. To what extent does the student select appropriate question forms to obtain specific pieces of information?

   b. To what extent does the student display a variety of question types?

   c. To what extent is the student able to ask questions in a socially acceptable manner without causing the speaker to feel annoyed?

3. Negation

   a. To what extent does the student use a high incidence of double negatives (e.g., I ain't got no book)?

   b. To what extent is the student able to say "No" or disagree appropriately?

4. Nonspecific Words

   a. To what extent does the student use a high frequency of low information words to describe events, persons, or actions, rather than using exact labels (e.g., using words such as "thing," "stuff," "someone," "anyone," "whatchamacallit")?

   b. To what extent does the student recognize the need to use more specific descripters in order for an unfamiliar listener to comprehend the message?

5. Figurative Language

   a. To what extent does the student use enough current slang and jargon of the adolescent culture to avoid being identified by the peer group as "different" based on use of figurative language (see also, "Assessment Strategies: Survival Language Skills")?

   b. To what extent does the student use idioms, metaphors, and other figurative language to entertain when appropriate?

6. Word Retrieval/Vocabulary

   a. To what extent does the student appear to search for words while talking (i.e., word retrieval problems)?

   b. To what extent does the student use strategies to self-cue when retrieving words?

   c. To what extent, if any, does lack of specific vocabulary items interface with word retrieval problems?

B. Paralinguistics

1. Vocalized Pause

   a. To what extent does the student use vocalized pauses (e.g., um, ah)? Is it distracting to the listener? Is it indicative of word retrieval problems?

   b. To what extent does the vocalized pause slow the rate of delivery? Is it slowed to a point where it is difficult for the listener to comprehend the spoken message?

2. Verbal Mazes

   a. To what extent do verbal mazes interfere with the listener's ability to comprehend spoken messages?

   b. To what extent does the student spontaneously recognize when he/she is engaged in a verbal maze and have strategies for revising the utterance?

   c. To what extent does the student begin almost all utterances with a false starter (e.g., "you know")?

C. Conversational Acts

1. Topic Shifts

   a. To what extent does the student initiate new topics when it is appropriate to do so?

b. To what extent is the student able to remain on a topic for an indefinite amount of time providing the topic is interesting to both conversational partners?

c. To what extent does the student provide the listener with cues when conversational topics are being shifted (i.e., use of transitional statements)?

d. To what extent is the student able to make the switch between speaker and listener roles during conversation? Is it done with ease, taking turns in an appropriate manner?

2. Interruption

a. To what extent does the student show occasional use of positive verbal reinforcement during the speaking turn of the conversational partner (e.g., saying "Uh-huh," "Mm," while the other person is speaking to indicate "I am understanding you")?

b. To what extent does the student show any verbal or nonverbal interruptions that indicate "I do not understand you" (e.g., "Huh?" or a frown)? If so, are they done in a way that does not annoy the listener?

c. To what extent does the student engage in negative interruptions during the speaking turn of the conversational partner (e.g., making distracting gestures or verbalizations)?

3. Functions

a. To what extent does the student use language to give information?

b. To what extent does the student use language to get information?

c. To what extent does the student use language to describe an ongoing event?

d. To what extent does the student use language to get a listener to feel, believe, or do something?

e. To what extent does the student use language to describe his/her own beliefs, feelings, etc.?

f. To what extent does the student use language to indicate a readiness for further communication?

87

g. To what extent does the student use language to problem solve?

h. To what extent does the student use language to entertain?

D. Qualitative Analysis

Lucas (1980) has posed additional questions that are not addressed above nor answered by our present standardized tests. She suggests questions that we find particularly applicable to adolescent language:

1. To what extent has the language sample contained objects, actions, and events in a variety of relationships?

2. To what extent has the student used a variety of forms to express a variety of functions?

3. To what extent has the student used utterances that are appropriate for the context?

4. To what extent has the student answered questions appropriately? To what extent has the student only responded, oblivious to question form?

5. To what extent has the student used the same construction repeatedly with some of the same lexical terms?

6. To what extent has the student performed a variety of speech acts?

7. To what extent has the student used a variety of terms to denote space, time, quantity, and/or quality?

E. Behavioral Observations

Lucas (1980) also suggested that the examiner ask the following types of behavioral observation questions to help determine the strategies being used by the student:

1. To what extent does the student observe the listener's face when in the speaker's role?

2. To what extent does the student appropriately respond verbally while engaged in another activity (i.e., can the student engage in another activity while talking)?

3. To what extent does the student's oral communication interfere negatively with reading and writing?

4. To what extent does the student use body movement to manipulate the environment? Students who rely on body movement to meet needs are having problems being effective communicators.

5. To what extent does the student use gestures or pantomime as a replacement for oral communication?

6. To what extent does the student verbalize more or less with different people in different situations?

IV. HOW TO ASSESS LANGUAGE PRODUCTION/CONVERSATIONAL SKILLS

A. Informal Procedures

1. Conversational Speech Samples

a. Obtain at least two five-minute samples of conversational speech in different settings with a minimum of 50 speaker turns. You may wish to tape additional minutes then eliminate the first few minutes of the analysis. Sample settings might include conversational speech with a friend, an unfamiliar peer of the same sex (or opposite sex), or a familiar adult of the same sex (or opposite sex). If at all possible, video record the conversations; second best is to audio record. Do not remain with the student unless you are the conversational partner. If assistance in topic generation is needed, suggest hobbies, after-school activities, or school/family routines.

b. Listen and critique initially for gross deviations from what you know to be "normal." Develop a "feel" for the conversation that took place.

c. Transcribe the entire sample (both conversational partners). Determine what your unit of measurement will be (e.g., Loban's communication unit). The L-B analysis described below is based on conversational units, the utterances of one conversational partner that continue until the other conversational partner initiates an independent utterance. An utterance may be defined as "any vocalization," thus making an independent utterance "any nonsimultaneous vocalization." (See page 106 for a sample transcription of normal adolescents.)

d. Analyze the sample using a system published in the literature or one that you have devised. Note that stages of linguistic development and mean length of utterance in morphemes are not appropriate criteria for analyzing the language of adolescents. Several possible analysis procedures are outlined below:

89

(1) Charlann Simon's Communicative Competence
    (1979)

Charlann Simon's clinician's model of expressive communicative competence can be a helpful source for analyzing conversational speech samples. The examiner can check the student's language/conversational skills against Simon's list of competent versus incompetent features of form, function, and style. Using a simple binary system of "yes - no" combined with qualitative statements, the examiner can have access to a fairly efficient analysis sytem. For example, the authors have adapted Simon's model of expressive communicative competence:

(a) Student uses flexible, precise vocabulary?
    ____Yes ____No

    Observations and Comments:_____

    _____

(b) Student has mastery of syntactics and morphological rules? ____Yes ____No

    Observations and Comments:_____

    _____

(c) Student uses complexity and a variety of syntactics? ____Yes ____No

    Observations and Comments:_____

    _____

(d) Student has mastery of irregular grammatical features? ____Yes ____No

    Observations and Comments:_____

    _____

(e) Student has mastery of tense reference and subject/verb agreement? ____Yes ____No

    Observations and Comments:_____

    _____

(f) Student uses clear noun referents?
    ____Yes ____No

    Observations and Comments:_____

    _____

(g) Student uses subordinators to relate
    ideas? ____Yes   ____No

    Observations and Comments: _____

    _____

The examiner could develop similar analysis
forms from Simon's categories of function and
style.

(2) Loban's Analysis of Transcripts (1976)

For a detailed description of Loban's Analysis
System, it is recommended the examiner refer to
Language Development: Kindergarten through
Grade 12, National Counsel of Teachers of Eng-
lish, 1111 Kenyon Road, Urbana, Illinois 61801.
Major components of his analysis sytem in-
clude the following:

(a) Communication Units -- Loban defined a
    communication unit as each independent
    clause with its modifier. The number of
    communication units was tabulated for
    the language sample and it was indicated
    that units fall into one of the follow-
    ing three categories:

    (i)   Independent grammatical predica-
          tions

    (ii) Answers to a question, provided the
          answers lack only the repetition
          of the question elements to satisfy
          their criterion of independent pre-
          dications.

    (iii) Words such as "yes" or "no" when
          given in answer to "yes-no" ques-
          tions.

(b) Counting Words -- Loban counted words with-
    in each communication unit. He computed
    average number of words per communication
    unit and used this measurement as a pri-
    mary tool of comparison among different
    grade levels.

(c) Mazes -- Using nonessential repetitions,
    making false starts, or becoming confused
    or tangled in words were counted as verbal
    mazes. Loban computed the total number
    of mazes per language sample and the

91

average number of words per maze. This measurement was also used as a basic comparison tool among students in different grade levels.

(d) Subordination -- Using a blue pencil, Loban underlined adjective, adverb, or noun phrases twice. Dependent clauses were enclosed in blue parentheses.

(e) Phonological Units -- Loban marked pauses or silences in the subject's speech. Clear-cut terminations of utterances were marked as were definite pauses and momentary silences.

(3) Larson-Boyce Analysis of Conversational Speech (Larson and Boyce, in preparation) (See Glossary for definition of terms.)

(a) Linguistic

(i) Sentences: Mark simple sentences with a blue dot. Mark complex sentences with a red dot. If the complex sentence is a "run-on" series of simple sentences conjoined with "and," put (R-O) above the red dot.

(ii) Features: Mark the following features as they occur within the student's conversational turns:

-- Question Forms

-- Negations

-- Figurative Language

-- Nonspecific Language

Count frequency of occurrence for each of the features (e.g., three instances of slang occurred in conversational unit number 3) and mark that number in the appropriate space on the data grid (see sample grid on the next page).

(iii) Word Retrieval: Count frequency of occurrence of word retrieval problems, but also qualitatively analyze the student's ability to use self-cues. If you are uncertain whether

92

CONVERSATIONAL UNITS

		1	2	3	4	5	6	7	8	9	10
SENTENCES:	Fragment										
	Simple										
	Complex										
	Run-On										
QUESTIONS:	Wh										
	Tag										
	Interrogative Reversal										
	Rising Intonation										
NEGATION:	Simple										
	Double										
FIGURATIVE LANGUAGE											
NONSPECIFIC LANGUAGE											
WORD RETRIEVAL											

the problem is one of word retrieval or lack of vocabulary, provide the student with a multiple choice of words. A student with word retrieval problems will be able to identify the desired word within the group presented. A student lacking vocabulary will not recognize the word even when presented.

(b) Paralinguistics

    (i) Mark vocalized pauses as they occur within the student's conversational turns. Count frequency of occurrence per unit and mark the appropriate grid space (see sample grid on the next page).

   (ii) Mark verbal mazes as they occur within the student's conversational turns. Count frequency of occurrence per unit and mark the appropriate grid space (see sample grid on the next page).

(c) Conversational Acts

    (i) Mark topic shifts that were made by the student. Determine whether they were related or unrelated. If unrelated, analyze whether a transition statement or gesture was used. Record data in the appropriate grid space (see sample grid on the next page).

   (ii) Mark verbal interruptions made by the student. Determine whether they were positive or negative. Record frequency of occurrence on the line between the two conversational units which encompass the interruption. (Remember that interruptions occur during the partner's turn, not within the student's conversational units.) (See sample grid on the next page.)

  (iii) Determine the overall function of the conversational unit. Record one function per unit in the appropriate grid space (see sample grid on the next page).

94

CONVERSATIONAL UNITS

		1	2	3	4	5	6	7	8	9	10
PARALINGUISTICS	Verbal Pause										
	Verbal Maze										
CONVERSATIONAL ACTS	Topic Shift: Related										
	Topic Shift: Unrelated										
	Transition: Present										
	Transition: Not Present										
	Interruptions: Positive										
	Interruptions: Negative										
	Functions:										
	--To give information										
	--To get information										
	--To describe an ongoing event										
	--To get listener to feel/ believe/do something										
	--To describe one's beliefs, feelings, etc.										
	--To indicate readiness for further communication										
	--To problem solve										
	--To entertain										
NONVERBAL COMMUNICATION	Gestures: Supportive										
	Gestures: Nonsupportive										
	Interruptions: Positive										
	Interruptions: Negative										

(d)   Nonverbal Communication

      (i)   Mark gestures made by the student during the conversational unit. Looking at the entire unit, determine whether the gestures were basically supportive of the verbal message or basically nonsupportive Keep in mind that nonsupportive gestures may or may not be inappropriate and/or distracting to the listener. Total frequency of gestures is not critical data to record. Each grid space will have one mark in either "Gestures - Supportive" or "Gestures - Nonsupportive" (see sample grid on page 95).

      (ii) Mark nonverbal interruptions made by the student during the speaking turn of the conversational partner. Determine whether they were positive or negative. Record frequency of occurrence on the line between the two conversational units which encompassed the interruption. (Remember that interruptions occur during the partner's turn, not within the student's conversational units.) (See sample grid on page 95.)

2.   Observational Scales

The following scales are informal in the sense that they do not place the student in a standardized test situation or they are completed by educators who rate spoken language performance noted during daily interactions.

a.   In Oral Proficiency Testing (Gary, Indiana, 1977) students are interviewed for approximately two minutes while they respond to four open-ended questions concerning educational and social matters. Interviews are recorded and scored by a team of three members, none of whom are presently teachers for the student. (In Gary, no team member is allowed to score students who are presently attending his/her home school.)

The following rating scale is used:

    4 - Moderately to Highly Proficient

    3 - Typically Proficient

    2 - Deficient to Moderately Deficient

    1 - Severely Deficient

In order to pass, a student must score a total of at least 24 points in these categories:

    i.   Articulation

   ii.   Pronounciation

  iii.   Verbal Utterances (talking without verbal crutches such as "you know," "and such")

   iv.   Rate

    v.   Word Usage (Standard grammatical form)

   vi.   Voice Quality

  vii.   Volume

 viii.   Sentence Structures

The student does not pass with scores below 3 in more than two categories. Informal but structural procedures such as this one are effective ways for "regular" educators to contribute to the assessment process and evaluate the overall nature of the student's language production.

b. A <u>teacher observation checklist</u> by Loban (1976) has been used effectively to assist in identifying and assessing language disordered students.

c. Backland, et al. (1982) recommended a <u>four-point rating scale</u> that assesses students' delivery, language, organization, and purpose. For example, in the language area, they proposed the following rating:

    4 - Speaker is consistently intelligible; always uses words and phrases and standard English, creating an impression of fluency.

3 - Speaker is generally intelligible, but shows occasional errors in standard English usage and some hesitation in choosing words and phrases.

2 - Speaker is moderately intelligible, but shows frequent errors in standard usage and much hesitation in choosing words and phrases.

1 - Speaker is barely intelligible; seldom uses words and phrases in standard English usage and shows stress in choosing words.

--- Did not respond

--- No opportunity to respond

Students who consistently rate at 1 and 2 are likely targets for intervention services.

d. Examiners can create <u>rating scales based upon</u> THEIR <u>particular needs</u>. Low ratings by other educators within the school will add information about the student's language and support for intervention services. Such rating scales can also serve as referral forms (see also, the example referral forms in the Delivery of Services section).

3. <u>Directed Verbalization</u>

Using tasks such as describing diagrams or multi-action pictures (see Assessment Strategies: Cognitive Skills), or talking about a specified topic, the examiner can systematically answer the questions in the previous Section III, "What to Assess," with the exception of those that require conversational speech. The examiner could also complete a rating scale such as those discussed previously, based upon the student's responses. The following types of directed verbalization tasks and example assessment activities are suggested for adolescent students.

a. Asking for and giving straightforward information

  i. Have the student direct a visitor to the school office.

  ii. Have the student direct an out-of-state tourist from the school to a motel.

98

iii.   Tell the ambulance driver how to reach the school or home.

iv.   Direct a person to the nearest entrance to the interstate highway.

v.   Explain to a new student the school dress code or some other regulation.

b.   Describing objects, events, experiences, and explaining a project.

i.   Have the student describe an event that he/she recently attended (e.g., a ball game, a party).

ii.   Have the student describe to someone else how to find a particular book from a number of books in a locker.

iii.   Have the student choose a topic on which to make a report. Urge the student to include a few details that can be written out in note form. Give the student overnight to prepare. The presentation should explain how a process, procedure, or mechanical feature functions. For example, it might explain a football game or the procedure for installing a tape deck in an automobile. The talk should be judged on the basis of organization, logic, and clarity of the oral presentation. Ideally, this presentation would be given to several people, not just to the examiner in isolation.

c.   Questioning another's viewpoint

i.   Have the student ask a question about someone's position regarding school policy or tradition.

ii.   Have the student question a fellow student's interpretation of a recent movie or television program.

iii.   Simulate a job interview in which the student is required to ask questions about the job.

iv.   Have the students question a teacher (or provide a simulated situation) about course requirements and the form and content of an upcoming examination.

99

v. Have the student ask questions to fill in information when incomplete messages are given (e.g., A parent needs to let a student know that his dental appointment has been changed. What information does the student need in order to complete the message?).

d. Speaking so one's listener understands the purpose

    i. Have the student talk with the teacher (or provide a simulated situation) to get information on a homework assignment or to question a grade.

    ii. Have the student use a telephone to find out if a store has a certain product.

    iii. Have the student get the number of a new family that has just moved into town.

    iv. Have the student introduce his/her parents (or provide a simulated situation) to a teacher or the principal.

    v. Have the student explain to a potential employer (or provide a simulated situation) what hours he/she has available for working.

e. Describing another's viewpoint or differences in opinion and expressing feelings to others

    i. Have the student describe the viewpoint of his/her parent(s) regarding a recent disagreement.

    ii. Have the student describe differences in opinion regarding the best rock group.

    iii. Have the student express satisfaction or dissatisfaction to an instructor (or in a simulated situation) about a class being taken.

    iv. Have the student express what he/she would say to a friend who has not done well in a class.

B. Formal Instruments

Few published tests exist solely for the purpose of assessing language production/conversational skills of adolescents. A number of tests are appropriate for all ages (e.g., Psycho-Educational Battery, 1977) and many contain only portions or sections that are useful. The following is a partial list of tests that the authors recommend for consideration. It is not intended to be an exhaustive listing of available resources. Keep in mind, too, that tests listed in other sections may be applicable to production analysis as well. The authors believe that formal tests are used primarily to confirm what you have already observed and/or documented through informal procedures.

1. Test of Adolescent Language
   (Hammill, et al., 1980)

   The TOAL has two subtests that are appropriate for language production assessment:

   a. "Speaking/Vocabulary" tests by giving a student a word to produce within a sentence.

   b. "Speaking/Grammar" tests by asking a student to repeat a sentence.

   Scaled scores are available for ages 11 years through 18 years, 5 months.

2. Clinical Evaluation of Language Functions
   (Semel and Wiig, 1980)

   The CELF has five subtests that focus upon production:

   a. "Producing Word Series" tests by naming the days of the week and the months of the year.

   b. "Producing Names on Confrontation" tests by naming the color and shape of a series of forms as rapidly as possible.

   c. "Producing Word Associations" tests by naming foods as quickly as possible, then animals.

   d. "Producing Model Sentences" tests by using a sentence repetition format.

   e. "Producing Formulated Sentences" tests by having a student produce a sentence containing a specified vocabulary word.

A supplementary subtest, "Producing Speech Sounds" is also available. A CELF "Advanced Level Screening Test" that includes language production items is also available. Norms are available through Grade 12.

3. Language Assessment Tasks
   (Kellman, Flood and Yoder, 1977)

   The LAT contains several subsections that would be appropriate to use: "Assessment of Production" and "Assessment of Communicative Function." "Assessment of Production" includes these applicable subtests:

   a. Articulation, which is tested only if necessary

   b. Voice/Fluency, which is completed in narrative fashion, if necessary

   c. Syntax, which is tested by:

      i. Taping and transcribing a language sample

      ii. Having the student produce a specified conjunction within a sentence

      iii. Obtaining a student's written language sample through a classroom teacher and comparing it to oral language

   d. Semantics, which is tested by:

      i. Vocabulary, having the students supply definitions for words

      ii. "Wh" questions, having the students ask about a picture until they determine what it is

   "Assessment of Communicative Function" is tested by questioning the student's teachers about the effectiveness of communication, using a list of specific functions as a guide.

4. Communication Competency Assessment Instrument
   (Rubin, 1982)

   This assessment instrument is based on minimal speaking and listening competencies for high school graduates. The instrument was originally developed to determine competence at the college level, but has recently included a format for high school students.

The instrument's procedures are identical, but the
questions are appropriate to the respective levels.
Students present a three-minute extemporaneous persuasive talk which is rated in identified skill areas.
They then listen to a videotaped lecture, and during
a dyadic interview, answer questions about the tape
and other experiences. This test may be appropriate
for late high school students.

5. Cognitive-Language-Communication Assessment Instrument
    (D.C. Everest Public Schools, Revised 1981)

    The CLC was developed by speech-language pathologists
    within a public school setting in response to the
    establishment of programs at the junior and senior
    high schools in the late 1970's. Several subsections
    are appropriate to mention here.

    a. "Oral Language-Expression" includes items that
        test linguistic structures (e.g., verb forms,
        inflectional endings, conjunctions); formulation
        of Wh-questions; use of basic vocabulary words;
        and use of ask/tell.

    b. "Pragmatics" include rating items such as eye
        contact, personal space, and turn taking in con-
        versation. The CLC also includes sections that
        assess other primary areas addressed in this
        manual.

6. Woodcock-Johnson Psycho-Educational Battery
    (Woodcock and Johnson, 1977)

    This instrument includes appropriate selected sub-
    tests in "Part One: Tests of Cognitive Ability" that
    require oral production responses:

    -- Picture vocabulary

    -- Memory for sentences

    -- Visual-Auditory learning

    -- Antonyms

    -- Synonyms

7. Detroit Tests of Learning Aptitude
    (Baker and Leland, 1967)

    This test includes appropriate selected subtests that
    require oral production responses:

-- Verbal opposites

-- Social adjustment A and B

-- Free association

-- Auditory attention span for related syllables

8. The Word Test
   (Jorgensen, et al., 1981)

   This test is normed only through age 12, making it appropriate for early adolescents but not directly applicable to older students. Its subtests require students to orally:

   -- Define words

   -- State multiple meanings for words

   -- Name antonyms and synonyms

   -- Explain semantic absurdities

   -- Make categorical associations

9. Let's Talk Inventory for Adolescents
   (Wiig, 1982)

   The purpose of the inventory is to elicit specific communication functions and speech acts relevant to social-oral communication contexts. It is suggested for use with students who are over 9 years of age to identify those with inadequate or delayed social communication skills. Field testing was completed with normal students from 7-14 years of age and with adolescents displaying language retardation. Speech act formulation and association tasks are tested for four communication functions:

   -- Ritualizing

   -- Informing

   -- Controlling

   -- Feeling

   Items probe for ability to formulate the intent and social register of speech acts in context with peers and with authority figures/adults. Sample items include, "Bob loves his cat Misty. Sometimes Bob tells Misty how much he loves her. What do you think Bob

says to Misty?" (formulation - feelings function)
and "Here are some more people. Who do you think
said: 'Why don't you open the door!' " (association -
controlling function).

V. SUMMARY

This section provides a rationale for assessing and teaching language production/conversational skills as well as data
on what to assess and how to assess this behavior. The authors
list available formal tests that might be used and present informal procedures for the reader's consideration.

SAMPLE TRANSCRIPT OF
CONVERSATIONAL SPEECH BETWEEN ADOLESCENTS
(Shelley and Kevin, both 15 years of age)

S.   They have this new thing at school, uh its for Valentines Day.
     It's a computer thing where you...they pick the ten most...
     Oh I forgot what the word is.

K.   Perfect couples?

S.   Yah, to see who you're matched up with?

K.   Uh huh

S.   And so we did that in Biology to figure out who hmm.

K.   Uh huh

S.   (laugh) all these stupid questions

K.   Yah, like what?

S.   What would you do on your date? Would you go to a movie or
     to a...

K.   Like dating game, right?

S.   Yah (laugh) they're real dumb.

K.   Who'd ya get?

S.   No, we have to pay a dollar to find out.

K.   Oh, did you pay?

S.   No, that's not until Valentines Day. It's just doing it
     before. They're just getting everybody to do it so...

K.   Oh. They're every-they're puttin everybody's name in but if
     you wanna find out you gotta pay the..... (pause) the eggs.

S.   Right. Everybody did it so I, it might be fun finding out.

K.   Are you gonna pay a dollar?

S.   I dunno, it'd be kinda neat just to find out who the...

K.   Watch it be Dan.

S.   (laugh) Yah, great.

K.   Brian Auckland

S. You bet (laugh).

S. It's in Biology the we haven't been doing anything cause of half the class was gone?

K. Uh huh

S. So it was we just sat there and watched a movie.

K. Uh huh

S. Tomorrow Walt Disney movie (laugh).

K. Oh, neat.

S. (laugh) Real fun.

K. Is it about Biology or is it just a Walt Disney?

S. 'Bout Mickey Mouse or something.

K. (laugh)

S. Mr. Kinches says we saw it in 7th grade, don't remember I was probly gone.

K. Yah ... They're looking in here. Bunch of janitors just walked by.

S. Oh, that's too bad. Let's see, down in weight training and conditioning we had this sub...

K. Ask questions.

S. What? We had this sub that I had in history class, oh, he's really, I don't like him at all, he's really a dick yah know? (laugh)

K. What'd he look like?

S. Um I dunno, he's not that bad looking but it was really funny he didn't remember me from history.

K. Yah?

S. So I was bein really nice to him. I was going "What's your name?" We were jogging for the minutes and I was talking to him as I go 'round and he'd say stuff to me and tell me what...

K. Jogging for five minutes? God that's real tough.

S. It was (laugh).

K. Well, hey, I know.

VI. ACTIVITIES

    A. What is happening in your state with regard to testing language production/conversational skills during grades 7-12?

        1.

        2.

        3.

    B. What kinds of speaking skills are deficient in your students (i.e., if you could change anything about the way your students presently speak, what would it be)?

        1.

        2.

        3.

    C. Whom do you consider to be a "good speaker" among the students you know?_____

What characteristics does that person(s) have that result in the label of "good speaker?"

        1.

        2.

What characteristics do you consider indicative of a "poor speaker?"

        1.

        2.

    D. List additional informal procedures and formal instruments you have found useful when assessing language production/ conversational skills in adolescents.

        1.

        2.

        3.

ASSESSMENT STRATEGIES: SURVIVAL LANGUAGE SKILLS

I. INTRODUCTION

A. Rationale for Assessing and Teaching Survival Language

Unfortunately, scant attention has been paid to the interpersonal and community living skills of adolescents despite
their functional relevance. The practical education of
adolescents, especially those with handicapping conditions,
has not been given the priority consideration it deserves.
Although it is possible for persons to survive "on the
streets" without the ability to read or write, it becomes
very difficult when they cannot speak or listen. As we
continuously strive toward normalizing the lives of all
handicapped individuals, the role of survival language
skills becomes paramount. Adolescents without an adequate
communication system will be unable to cope in our society.

B. Definition of Survival Language

Adults can examine their own lives to recognize the survival language skills they need every day. These are
skills that they must have to function successfully and
independently in their families, communities, and jobs
whether they are inside or outside the home.

C. Types of Survival Language Skills

Survival language skills can be divided into two main
categories each preceded by certain prerequisite concepts
and operations:

1. Situational language skills include comprehension and
   production of language necessary to survive a specific experience such as shopping in a supermarket,
   filling a prescription at the drugstore, eating in a
   restaurant, or buying a garment in a clothing store.

2. Multi-situational language skills cross a number of
   specific experiences and would be used in all of
   them. For example, appropriate use of money would be
   needed in all the situations cited in the examples
   above. Other examples include reading warning signs
   and labels, telling time, and using jargon/slang.

3. Prerequisite skills can be determined for all survival language skills. Most survival language skills
   rely on a firm foundation of spatial, quantitative,
   and temporal concepts. They often require basic cognitive operations such as classification, conservation,
   and causality.

II. ADOLESCENTS AS SURVIVAL LANGUAGE USERS

Each individual assumes various roles in order to fully function in our society. Valletutti and Bender (1982) have done
extensive curriculum development based upon a functional
approach to teaching. They have outlined the following roles
as ones essential to daily living:

A. Residing in a home

B. Learning in traditional and nontraditional school settings

C. Participating in the community

D. Being a consumer of goods and services

E. Working

F. Participating in leisure experiences

Each of these roles demands certain survival language skills.
These roles will be used as guidelines for questions asked in
the next section. After each question, readers may want to
indicate if it is primarily a situational survival language
skill (S) or a multi-situational skill (M-S).

III. WHAT TO ASSESS IN SURVIVAL LANGUAGE SKILLS

The following data is drawn from writings by Valletutti and
Bender (1982) and Bender and Valletutti (1982):

A. The Role of Resident in a Home

    1. To what extent does the student identify words and
       other symbols necessary for independent functioning
       in the home? Examples follow:

       a. Can the student turn on the desired burner after
          locating the appropriate dial or button that
          regulates the burner?

       b. Can the student select the desired setting on a
          toaster?

       c. Can the student prepare snacks, parts of meals,
          and complete meals following recipe directions
          and using measuring spoons and measuring cups?

       d. Can the student select desired food items from
          the name on package labels?

       e. Can the student open a food package by following
          directions printed on its label?

f. Can the student obey warnings found on household cleaning products?

g. Can the student set a thermostat for different times and different weather conditions?

h. Can the student review radio and television schedules and select desired programs?

i. Can the student follow washing and dry cleaning instructions found on clothing labels?

j. Can the student use grooming items according to directions printed on the labels?

k. Can the student determine how to wash or dry a load of laundry based upon the instructions given on the appliances?

2. To what extent does the student perform diverse oral or written tasks allowing him/her to function independently in the home? Examples follow:

a. Can the student write and interpret simple notes and messages for members of the household?

b. Can the student note key dates and appointments in a personal calendar?

c. Can the student relay greeting cards or use another way to communicate with relatives and friends?

3. To what extent does the student perform mathematical operations necessary for functioning independently in the home? Examples follow:

a. Can the student set the timer and/or heating level on the stove?

b. Can the student check sale expiration dates on packages or containers of food?

c. Can the student set an alarm clock, digital clock, or clock-radio to a desired wake-up time?

d. Can the student take over-the-counter medicines in dosages and at times recommended for adults?

e. Can the student check electric, gas, and/or water meter readings to confirm official meter readings on utility bills?

B. The Role of Student in Traditional and Nontraditional School Settings

1. To what extent does the student identify words and symbols found in the school in order to function independently? Examples follow:

   a. Can the student obey signs and directions on school buses and outside the school building?

   b. Can the student locate classrooms, offices, and other areas from names and numbers printed on doors and on signs placed near doorways?

   c. Can the student follow a class and activity schedule as it appears on his/her personal schedule card?

   d. Can the student locate restrooms from names printed on doors or signs placed near doorways?

   e. Can the student locate his/her personal locker and/or gym locker?

   f. Can the student use an electronic calculator to perform simple computations?

   g. Can the student follow written directions found throughout the school environment (or devise a strategy to have them read) and complete assignments as specified?

   h. Can the student locate key words on school-related forms and provide the requested information?

   i. Can the student locate important information on written announcements or in oral announcements and respond appropriately to the information and special requests?

2. To what extent does the student perform diverse oral or written tasks that will allow him/her to function independently in school? Examples follow:

   a. Can the student record relevant notes during class session?

   b. Can the student supply answers on written quizzes and examinations or have arrangements made to take tests orally?

   c. Can the student comprehend and produce enough slang so that communication with peers is not impaired?

112

3. To what extent does the student perform necessary mathematical operations so that he/she can function independently in school? Examples follow:

   a. Can the student unlock a combination lock on his/her school locker?

   b. Can the student move a specified number of places on a game board, tally scores, and carry out other mathematical computations during games?

   c. Can the student keep scheduled appointments with school personnel?

   d. Can the student locate the scores of "Home" and "Visitor" teams during sporting events and determine who is leading and by what amount?

   e. Can the student put the exact amount of change in a vending machine or put in more than the exact change and verify the correctness of the change received?

C. The Role of Participant in the Community

1. To what extent does the student identify words and symbols in the community in order to function independently? Examples follow:

   a. Can the student locate public rest rooms, public telephones, and mailbox pick-up sites?

   b. Can the student use a pay telephone?

   c. Can the student identify and use the correct amount of stamps to mail letters, greeting cards, and postcards?

   d. Can the student operate vending machines to obtain desired items?

   e. Can the student order meals from a restaurant menu?

   f. Can the student order a meal from a cafeteria or fast food restaurant bulletin board or directory?

   g. Can the student find a location by street signs, buildings, and/or house numbers?

   h. Can the student locate a specific room, apartment, or office from directional signs, numbers, and/or letters on the doors?

i. Can the student move about the community obey-
    ing warning signs and avoiding places designated
    as "dangerous?"

j. Can the student avoid entering doorways in build-
    ings designated as "no entry" or "authorized per-
    sonnel only?"

k. Can the student use a map to find his/her way
    around the community?

l. Can the student use maps to travel by bus, sub-
    way, or other mass transit vehicles?

m. As a driver, can the student obey symbols within
    the car or on traffic and parking signs?

n. Can the student operate self-service elevators
    at various places within the community?

o. Can the student obtain information of interest
    from local newspapers?

p. Can the student determine time by observing
    clocks and electronic time signs placed in build-
    ings in the community?

q. Can the student determine the temperatures by
    observing electronic temperature signs placed on
    buildings?

2. To what extent does the student perform various oral
   and written tasks so that he/she can function independently in the community? Examples follow:

   a. Can the student fill out and sign orders, requests,
       and application forms (e.g., job applications,
       order forms in catalog stores, deposit and with-
       drawal slips, and credit card application forms)?

   b. Can the student sign petitions and fill out sur-
       veys?

3. To what extent does the student perform the necessary
   mathematical operations in order to function independently in the community? Examples follow:

   a. Can the student pay for meals at restaurants and
       cafeterias?

   b. Can the student use signs on doors and windows,
       identify store and office hours, and plan to
       arrive and leave those businesses according to
       this information?

114

c. Can the student find residences 'and businesses or specific apartment numbers by number sequences appearing on surrounding houses?

d. Can the student estimate the amount of time needed to meet bus, train, subway, or airline schedules?

e. Can the student estimate the amount of time needed to arrive at businesses, restaurants, or other agencies after opening time or before closing time?

D. The Role of Consumer of Goods and Services

1. To what extent does the student identify words and other symbols that will allow him/her to function independently as a consumer of goods and services? Examples follow:

    a. Can the student prepare a shopping list and purchase the food on that list using the store directory when necessary?

    b. Can the student review the cost of desired food items at different stores and buy items where they are most economical?

    c. Can the student locate serving and portion information on food packages and buy the size and/ or number of packages needed for meals?

    d. Can the student compare the accuracy of store receipts with purchased items?

    e. Can the student compare the size and price of various over-the-counter drugs and medications and purchase the one(s) appropriate to his/her needs?

    f. Can the student differentiate medications to be applied externally from those to be taken internally?

    g. Can the student check clothing prices at different stores and buy needed items where they are most economical?

    h. Can the student locate laundromats and dry cleaners to take clothing to be washed and cleaned?

i. Can the student compare prices of furniture and appliances at different stores and buy needed items where they are most economical?

j. Can the student identify and observe warning signs on appliances?

k. Can the student identify signs and rebuses found in community places that announce the cost of admission?

l. Can the student identify various coins and denominations of bills and use these to pay for goods and services?

m. Can the student draw a check to pay for goods and services?

n. Can the student review warranties that accompany tools, materials, and other products?

o. Can the student identify information contained in mortgages and leases?

p. Can the student review the information on tax forms and arrange for them to be completed and filed on time?

q. Can the student review brochures, letters, and requests for fund raising organizations?

2. To what extent does the student perform diverse oral and written tasks in order to function independently as a consumer of goods and services? Examples follow:

a. Can the student write a letter of complaint, or deliver the complaint orally, relevant to consumer problems?

b. Can the student write or verbalize a request for consumer information?

c. Can the student fill out the forms necessary to open savings and checking accounts?

d. Can the student fill out various consumer-related application forms (e.g., application for a driver's license, a product warranty form, an application for a bank or credit union loan)?

e. Can the student draw up a weekly and monthly budget?

3. To what extent does the student perform necessary mathematical operations in order to function independently as a consumer of goods and services? Examples follow:

   a. Can the student estimate the cost of food and household products in his/her shopping basket to determine whether there is sufficient money to pay the bill?

   b. Can the student count change and verify its accuracy?

   c. Can the student buy desired clothing items after reviewing various size designations on tags and labels?

   d. Can the student compute the price of a sale item by subtracting a percentage discount?

   e. Can the student estimate the total cost of an item by including applicable sales tax and manufacturer's rebates?

   f. Can the student verify the accuracy of bank, store, or other monthly statements?

E. The Role of Worker

Bender and Valletutti (1982) stated that individuals who have work skills may not always possess job-seeking skills. They fail to obtain employment because they experience difficulty with the interview process and in completing job application forms. Basic work skills include applying for work, getting ready, going to work, following work rules, using interpersonal skills, managing work breaks, and applying for compensation. In addition, Bender and Valletutti have provided information about specific skills needed for entry level jobs in the 10 major occupational clusters: construction, health occupations, graphics and communication media, food preparation and service, manufacturing, clothing and textile, automotive and power service, office and business occupations, agriculture and natural resources, and distribution.

Specific jobs within these clusters might include janitor, hospital maid, printing press operator, busboy, welder, launderer, motorcycle mechanic, file clerk, logger, and cashier.

1. To what extent does the student identify words and other symbols so that he/she can function independently as a worker? Examples follow:

a. Can the student locate the Help Wanted section of newspapers and identify job offerings appropriate to his/her interests, needs and skills?

b. Can the student identify the skills required in special job clusters?

c. Can the student obtain a job application form and identify key words which request personal data information?

d. Can the student review job-related brochures and forms included in employee benefit packages (i.e., medical insurance, pension information, holiday schedules)?

e. Can the student identify time intervals on clocks and watches to be prepared to leave for work on time?

f. Can the student meet buses, car pools, and shuttle services after reviewing departure schedules?

g. Can the student locate the number of his/her employer in a personal telephone directory and call that person if unable to report to work?

h. Can the student follow directions on the time clock and time card and verify the time card after punching in and out?

i. Can the student follow directions and safety instructions on flammable and other dangerous substances with which he/she works?

j. Can the student follow the operating and safety instructions for tools, appliances, and machinery used on the job?

k. Can the student review work memos and appropriately share key information found on them?

l. Can the student check the gross amount of his/her paycheck and compare it to the time worked and rate of pay?

2. To what extent does the student perform diverse oral and written tasks so that he/she can function independently as a worker? Examples follow:

a. Can the student complete all required job-related forms such as work permits, social security applications, and tax withholding forms?

b. Can the student write simple notes or verbally communicate to supervisors the need for personal leaves and other special requests?

3. To what extent does the student perform necessary mathematical operations in order to function independently as a worker? Examples follow:

a. Can the student follow a daily wake-up schedule from the estimated time needed to leave for work?

b. Can the student count out a number of objects requested by a co-worker or predetermined number such as one in an assembly line task?

c. Can the student measure and cut required lengths and widths of various materials?

F. The Role of Participant in Leisure Experiences

1. To what extent does the student identify words and other symbols in order to function independently in leisure experiences? Examples follow:

a. Can the student follow instruction booklets for playing and scoring games?

b. Can the student identify suits and numbers in a standard deck of cards?

c. Can the student follow directions and rules for outdoor sporting and camping activities?

d. Can the student review directions included in model and craft kits and materials?

2. To what extent does the student perform diverse oral and written tasks so that he/she can function independently in leisure experiences? Examples follow:

a. Can the student write and/or construct words in knowledge and word games?

b. Can the student write for, or orally request, reservations for hotel rooms, concerts, or sports events?

c. Can the student fill out registration or check-in forms at hotels or resorts?

d. Can the student write friendly letters or make phone calls to friends and relatives?

3. To what extent does the student perform necessary mathematical operations so that he/she can function independently in leisure experiences? Examples follow:

   a. Can the student record and tally scores obtained in games and determine the winner and order of finish?

   b. Can the student identify the face value of cards and play his/her hand on that basis?

   c. Can the student total the number rolled on dice or spaces moved on a game board?

   d. Can the student determine time elapsed in activities involving speed and/or time periods?

   e. Can the student determine the cost of participating in various recreational activities?

IV. HOW TO ASSESS SURVIVAL LANGUAGE SKILLS

Throughout this section, it is critical to remember that what we are assessing and how, focuses upon the language underlying daily living tasks, not on performance of those tasks per se. For example, one of the questions above asked whether a student could operate a washer and dryer. More precisely, the concern would focus on whether that student had the necessary vocabulary to succeed in operating the washer. For example, did the student understand the concepts of "normal cycle," "prewash cycle," and "delicate cycle?" Did the student understand the difference between water levels and water temperature? Keeping in mind this distinction between necessary survival language versus the actual survival task, the following "How to Assess" suggestions are made.

A. Informal Procedures

Given real or simulated situations, the student is asked to role play or explain an appropriate response to the examiner. In some cases, the student may be asked to provide definitions. In other cases, such as schedules and graphs, the student may be asked to make interpretations. If initial assessment time is limited, the examiner may wish to study only multi-situational survival language tasks.

The following informal assessment tasks may be some of the first the examiner would wish to use with the student:

1. Money: Simulate a situation in which the student is expected to make a purchase. Assess whether the student can check the price of the item, estimate the total price (including sales tax), pay for the purchase in an appropriate manner, and verify the accuracy of change returned.

2. Time: Have the student perform a variety of real or simulated tasks involving temporal concepts. Suggested assessment activities include reading the clock, estimating the amount of time passed since the beginning of the assessment session, estimating the time it would take to complete various activities, and planning a shopping trip according to the constraints of business hours, assigning a specified number of errands.

3. Warnings and Informational Signs: The examiner is encouraged to present actual reproductions of warnings and informational signs common to the community where the student lives. A number of commercial publishers have now printed commercial signs available for classroom use. When using the signs for assessment purposes, evaluate the student's ability to understand the sign once it is decoded rather than the ability to read the sign per se.

4. Messages: Write or obtain messages about meetings or other events and assess the student's ability to comprehend the message and/or relay it to another person. For example: Mrs. Walters would like to pick up her daughter, Brenda, from school at 3:30 on December 3rd. She will meet her at the southeast entrance to the school building.

   Evaluate whether the student can transmit the content of the message verbally. Assessment can also include deleting portions of a message such as the date or a name, and asking the student to determine what information is missing that is critical for the message to make sense.

5. Slang/Jargon: Present statements or questions to the student that incorporate current slang/jargon used by other students in the school. Note ability to comprehend the utterances. Simulate a situation(s) in which the student is required to produce slang (e.g., describe a new student, a good-looking boy/girl, to your friend).

6. Prerequisite Skills: To ascertain whether the student has necessary prerequisite skills, the following assessment suggestions may be utilized:

a. A test of basic concepts (e.g., Test of Basic Concepts, 1971) may be used as a reference point for necessary vocabulary comprehension.

The authors hasten to add that if such a test is to be applied to junior or senior high school students, the concepts from the test could be used, but not the actual format. Rather, it is suggested that activities be appropriately modified for secondary level students.

b. Informal cognitive tasks such as those presented by Copeland (1974) will ascertain whether the student is "stuck" at some point in the concrete operational period (see also Assessment Strategies: Cognitive Skills section).

c. Lists such as the 100 Most Important Words (Horn, 1924) and the Dolch Basic 220 Word List (Dolch, 1949) provide an excellent starting point for informal assessment of basic requisite vocabulary needed for survival language skills.

B. Formal Instruments

Virtually no formal instruments are available for the assessment of survival language skills. A number of social maturity scales have been available for many years (e.g., Vineland Social Maturity Scale, 1965) although these instruments have not focused very specifically on multi-situational language skills such as the ones cited above. The formal instrument that surpasses all others at this point, with regard to assessment of survival language skills, is the Inventory of Essential Skills (Brigance, 1981). His extensive inventory includes sections such as measurements, health and safety, vocations, money and finance, travel and transportation, and food and clothing. Within these sections, specific subtests such as the following are completed: converting units of time, reading medicine labels, applying for social security numbers, reading "Help Wanted" advertisements, making change, following bus schedule and map routes, applying food preparation vocabulary, and reading clothing labels. Complete use of these sections within the Inventory of Essential Skills would provide the examiner with a wealth of knowledge about the survival language skills of the adolescent. It can also be noted that the Inventory of Essential Skills includes a multitude of personal rating scales to be completed by the individual who is being assessed. For example, there is a "job interview preparation rating scale," a "responsibility and self-discipline rating scale," and a "health practices and attitude rating scale."

V. SUMMARY

This section provides a rationale for assessing and teaching survival language skills as well as data on what to assess and how to assess this behavior. The authors list available formal tests that might be used and present informal procedures for the reader's consideration.

VI. ACTIVITIES

A. What is happening in your state with regard to testing of survival language skills during grades 7-12?

   1.

   2.

   3.

B. What kinds of survival language skills are deficient in your students?

   1.

   2.

   3.

C. Whom do you consider to be a "good survival language user" among the students you know?_____

   What characteristics does that person(s) have that result in the label of "good survival language user?"

   1.

   2.

   What characteristics do you consider to be indicative of a "poor survival language user?"

   1.

   2.

D. List additional informal procedures and formal instruments you have found useful when assessing survival language skills in adolescents.

   1.

   2.

   3.

ASSESSMENT STRATEGIES: EDUCATIONAL SYSTEM

I. INTRODUCTION

   A. Rationale for Assessing the Educational System

      1. It is conceivable that the "language problem" is
          within the educational system and not within the
          student. Assessing the education system will assist
          in identifying where the problem originates.

      2. It is possible that the primary problem is the stu-
          dent's lack of motivation. The "How to Assess"
          section that follows will assist the examiner in
          identifying students who are not motivated.

      3. In some cases, the intervention program designed
          for a language disordered adolescent will require
          modification of existing curriculum. In order to
          make that determination, the current program needs
          to be examined.

   B. Definition of Educational System

      Specifically, the authors are concerned with the curri-
      culum, as defined by the following components:

      1. The scope and sequence of skills taught

      2. The primary textbook used within each subject area

      3. The language of instruction used within the class-
          room setting

      4. The visual displays used such as charts, graphs,
          and maps

      5. The multimedia presentations used such as movies,
          videotapes, and television

      6. Any supplemental material such as workbooks and work-
          sheets

II. WHAT TO ASSESS IN THE EDUCATIONAL SYSTEM

    The effectiveness of language in the educational system can be
    evaluated by considering two basic facets:

    A. The language of instruction of the educators (Educators'
        language per se is not assessed, but rather the ability
        of the student to comprehend what is being said in the
        classroom and to interact verbally with the teacher.)

B. The language inherent in the curriculum content

III. <u>HOW TO ASSESS THE EDUCATIONAL SYSTEM</u>

The authors have developed a suggested format for curriculum
analysis entitled <u>CALI: Curriculum Analysis - Language of
Instruction</u>. It is designed to look at a specific subject
area, assessing both the language of the textbook and the
language used in the classroom. The CALI is outlined on the
following pages.

CALI: Curriculum Analysis - Language of Instruction

Date(s) of Analysis:_____   Examiner Completing Analysis:_____

Student: _____   Course: _____

Grade Level:_____   Instructor: _____

I.   **TEXTBOOK ANALYSIS** (Use the primary text from the course.)

   A. **Identifying Information**

   1. Title:_____
   2. Author(s):_____
   3. Copyright: _____
   4. Year Adopted by School:_____
   5. Readability Level:_____
   6. Topic Arrangement (Check one):
       ____Sequential - Independence Among Topics
       ____Spiral - Dependence Among Topics

   B. **Student Familiarity with Textbook**

   Check which of the following features are included in the textbook. For any that are present, check whether the student can locate these features upon request and state when they are used:

Check if Present:	Features	Can the Student locate the feature?	When is the feature used?
_____1.	Table of Contents	____yes ____no	_____
_____2.	Index	____yes ____no	_____
_____3.	Glossary	____yes ____no	_____
_____4.	Appendix	____yes ____no	_____
_____5.	Bibliography	____yes ____no	_____
_____6.	Unit or Chapter Objectives	____yes ____no	_____
_____7.	Review Questions and/or Practice Exercises	____yes ____no	_____
_____8.	Italicization of Words (Varying Print Styles)	____yes ____no	_____
_____9.	Graphic Aids (Charts, Tables, Graphs, Maps)	____yes ____no	_____

Larson, V. and Boyce, N. © 1983

C. Student Comprehension of the Textbook

Prior to involving the student, select a segment of the textbook no longer than three pages in length. As the examiner, identify the main idea within the selected passage and relevant supporting details.

Summarize this information below:

Page(s):_____

Main Idea:_____

_____

_____

Relevant Details:_____

_____

_____

_____

With the student present, deliver the information above using an informal lecture style. Upon completion of the delivery ask the student to cite the main idea. Then formulate two questions that refer to the relevant supporting details. Transcribe your questions and the student's responses exactly as they occurred. The student may take notes.

1. What was the main idea?_____

_____

2. Relevant Detail Question #1
   (Record exact wording of question):

   _____

   Student's response:_____

3. Relevant Detail Question #2

   _____

   Student's Response:_____

Repeat with additional passages, if desired and/or necessary.

Now answer the following questions:

1. Did the student's main idea match the one you identified? _____yes _____no
2. Did the student's relevant supporting details match the ones you identified?
   _____yes _____no
3. Did the student indicate verbally or nonverbally any words that were not understood?
   _____yes _____no
   If "yes", list them:_____

   _____

II. CLASSROOM ANALYSIS

A. Student's Comprehension of Lecture/Instructions

Arrange a 5-10 minute period in which you can observe the student in the classroom and at the same time listen to the instructor give information or instructions using a lecture style. Take notes on main ideas and supporting details as if you were a student. During your next session with the student, compare notes for the time you observed. Ask the student to identify the main idea and supporting details using his/her notes.

1. What was the main idea presented (or sequence of instructions?)_____
_____

2. What were the relevant supporting ideas?_____
_____

Now, answer the following questions:
1. Did the student's main idea match the one you identified?

_____yes _____no

2. Did the student's relevant supporting details match the ones you identified?

_____yes _____no

3. Did the student indicate verbally or nonverbally any words that were not understood?

_____yes _____no

If "yes", list them:_____
_____

B. Student's Comprehension of Tests/Evaluations

Obtain a recent test or other evaluation tool administered to the student. With the student present, ask the following questions:

1. What questions were most difficult to answer?
_____

Why were they more difficult?_____
_____

2. What vocabulary items were unfamiliar?
_____
_____
_____

3. How well did you prepare for this test? (circle one)

----+-------------------+-------------------+-------------------------+----------------------------+----------

Not at all   Some   Enough   More than   A great amount
                                                     usual

4. Using the taxonomy from Benjamin Bloom*, what level(s) of thinking was required most often during this test?

_____ Memory   _____ Analysis
_____ Translation   _____ Synthesis
_____ Interpretation   _____ Evaluation
_____ Application

*Bloom, B., Ed., *Taxonomy of Educational Objectives, The Classification of educational goals: Handbook I: Cognitive Domain. New York: Longman, Inc. 1956.*

C. **Instructor Observation: Communication in the Classroom.**

Request participating instructors to complete the observation form attached to the end of this curriculum analysis and return it to the examiner.

1. Total number of points scored:_____(A)

2. Total number of "NA" (not appropriate) x5:_____(B)

3. Subtract "NA" points from 50:_____(C)

4. Compute percentage by $\dfrac{(A)}{(C)}$ x 100 = _____%

III. **STUDENT ANALYSIS**

Using the scales provided, have the student respond to the following pairs of words as they relate to a particular subject in the curriculum. Read and interpret the words for the student, if necessary. Direct the student to circle the point on the scale between each word pair that describes how he/she feels toward the subject. These feelings are based on the total course. (i.e., textbook and classroom).

Subject in the Curriculum:_____

Good	Clear	Important	Interesting	Complicated	Useless	Meaningful	
—	—	—	—	—	—	—	
—	—	—	—	—	—	—	
—	—	—	—	—	—	—	
—	—	—	—	—	—	—	
—	—	—	—	—	—	—	Neutra
—	—	—	—	—	—	—	
—	—	—	—	—	—	—	
—	—	—	—	—	—	—	
—	—	—	—	—	—	—	
Bad	Confusing	Unimportant	Uninteresting	Simple	Useful	Meaningless	

Instructor Observation: Communication in the Classroom

Instructor's Name:_____ Student's Name:_____

Date:_____ Course:_____

When assigning values to the communication behavior below, use a "NA" (not appropriate) for items that you cannot evaluate.

---------- 1 ---------- ---------- 2 ---------- ---------- 3 ---------- ---------- 4 ---------- ---------- 5 ----------
Inadequate   Minimally   "Borderline"   Adequate   Above
              Adequate   Adequate

Rating:

_____1. Ability to follow a sequence of directions (3 or more) given in a classroom.

_____2. Ability to comprehend main ideas presented during lectures.

_____3. Ability to comprehend the vocabulary of the course.

_____4. Ability to participate in classroom discussion and make verbal contributions to the class.

_____5. Ability to use questions to find specific additional information or to clarify previous information.

_____6. Ability to produce statements and questions that are intelligible, organized, and appropriate to the situation.

_____7. Ability to carry on a conversation with other students and/or instructor.

_____8. Ability to engage in problem solving/thinking/reasoning required in course.

_____9. Voice characteristics appropriate to one's sex and age.

_____10. Fluency in using the language; freedom from excessive verbal mazes, repetitions, and/or struggling to find the right word (i.e., word retrieval problem).

Please list any additional comments pertinent to this student's communication in your classroom.

Larson, V. and Boyce, N. © 1983

Thinking Ink Publications

IV. <u>SUMMARY</u>

In order to fully determine the nature of the suspected language disorder, it is critical to assess the educational system. The <u>CALI: Curriculum Analysis - Language of Instruc-
tion</u> was developed by the authors to focus on language aspects
of textbooks and educators and on the attitudes of students
toward particular subjects.

V. ACTIVITIES

A. Critique the <u>CALI: Curriculum Analysis - Language of Instruction</u> in regard to its strengths and weaknesses.

Strengths: 1.

2.

3.

Weaknesses: 1.

2.

3.

B. What additional information do you view as critical to obtain during assessment of the educational system with regard to the textbook, educator, or student?

1.

2.

3.

ASSESSMENT STRATEGIES: ENVIRONMENTAL CONDITIONS

I. INTRODUCTION

A. Rationale for Assessing Environmental Conditions

Each student is a part of some family unit that provides
the foundation for experiences, beliefs, and values.
Likewise, each student has a surrounding peer group that
is influential during adolescent years. Typically, more
attention and time is focused upon family and friend concerns by the language disordered adolescent than upon
academic concerns. Because close social contacts form
the basis of the student's stability and self-esteem,
it is imperative that we include the family and peer
group within the assessment process.

B. Definition of Environmental Conditions

Environmental conditions that are particular concerns to
us include the language systems of both the student's
family and peers and their attitudes toward the person
with a language disorder.

II. WHAT TO ASSESS IN ENVIRONMENTAL CONDITIONS

A. Family

It is important to assess the family's language style to
determine if the student's linguistic behavior is unique
or part of the family's communication system. We can
then determine if we are dealing with a communication disorder or a difference. The intervention protocol will
vary dependent upon this determination. We also need to
assess the family's attitude toward their child's communication behavior.

B. Peers

Since there is a paucity of data on normal communication
development, assessing the peer's language system is
extremely important for determining what is normal speech-
language-communication behavior for this age group. Also,
by analyzing the peer's language system it may be possible
to determine how the peers may be requiring the student
with a language disorder to comprehend or produce language
(i.e., Valspeak, idiomatic expressions, slang, etc.).

III. **HOW TO ASSESS ENVIRONMENTAL CONDITIONS**

   A. <u>Use of an Interview With the Family</u>

Both the family's communication style and attitudes might be appraised from an interview. According to Emerick (1969), an interview "....is a purposeful exchange of meanings between two persons, a directed conversation that proceeds in an orderly fashion to obtain data, to convey certain information, and to provide release and support." The following recommendations for conducting the interview are advised:

1. The speech-language pathologist should conduct the interview in an atmosphere that is comfortable and purposeful.

2. Questions should be asked in an open-ended manner, encouraging the family to share information for the good of the student.

3. Any necessary note taking should be done in a non-distracting manner.

4. When attempting to obtain information or provide release and support, the speech-language pathologist should listen first, then speak.

   a. Be an active/therapeutic listener who tries to understand what the parents perceive as the problem, what they feel about the problem, and what their message means.

   b. As an active listener, you do not evaluate or advise the parents at this time.

5. When conveying information to the parent, it is important that the speech-language pathologist present information clearly and concisely without using professional jargon.

6. ALL important information should be transmitted to the parent orally and in writing. The written word remains long after the spoken word.

7. Once an interview has been conducted, the speech-language pathologist should analyze the information for major themes in the parents' presentation, association of ideas, inconsistencies, and possible omissions.

8. A constructive interview should yield sufficient
    data to analyze and determine the parents' linguis-
    tic style and their feelings and attitudes toward
    their child's language disorder.

B. Use of Observation With Peers

The peers of the student with a language disorder should
be observed to determine the requirements they are making
regarding production and comprehension of language (i.e.,
slang, jargon, idiomatic expressions).

1. Observe both formal and informal speaking situations.

2. Record significant details regarding the demands they
    place on their peers to comprehend and produce the
    language.

IV. SUMMARY

The assessment strategy is not fully completed until consideration is given to the family and peers of the student with
a language disorder. In some cases, the student may actually
have a language difference rather than a disorder which would
have a drastic impact on the intervention strategies provided.
It is also important to assess attitudes and feelings toward
the student with a language disorder.

V. ACTIVITIES

A. List additional interview strategies that you have found useful with families of language disordered students. (If you have not participated in interviews, what skills do you feel you would need to develop in order to successfully interview parents?)

   1.

   2.

   3.

B. List situations in which you could observe various peer groups of your adolescent clients.

   1.

   2.

   3.

INTERVENTION

OVERVIEW OF THE INTERVENTION PROCESS FOR ADOLESCENTS

I. ## INTRODUCTION

During the assessment process we examined whether the problem
was within the student, the educational system, or the environmental conditions. Because problems may be identified in
any or all of these places, the intervention model purposely
addresses strategies to use with all three. Figure 2 illustrates the global intervention model the authors suggest for
use with adolescents.

II. ## GENERAL INTERVENTION PRINCIPLES

Just as basic principles of assessment are important to consider so, too, are general intervention principles. Many of
the principles discussed for assessment also apply to the
intervention process (see also Delivery of Services, II. D.
Intervention section). The authors suggest that these additional principles be considered:

A. ### Determine the Purpose of Intervention

Many students with language disorders will have multiple
problems and it is crucial to prioritize what will receive
attention first. This is not an arbitrary decision on the
part of the educator; rather, the decision process allows
the student primary input in ranking needed skills in the
order of importance. In essence, students determine what
is most critical for their particular lives; they are not
told what to do. Until students recognize their problems,
and take ownership of them, they will not be motivated to
make behavioral changes.

B. ### Establish Responsibility for the Language Disorder

There needs to be no "hidden agenda" when providing intervention services for adolescents. Preschoolers and elementary students frequently do not know what the terminal
objectives are during their remediation. With adolescents,
it is important to establish that they are responsible
for taking care of their language disorder, not the involved professionals. The students are the ones who stand
to lose if they do not develop appropriate communication
skills. Contracts between students with language disorders and educators have often been helpful in establishing this sense of responsibility. If the adolescent does
not want responsibility, denies the existence of a problem, and/or remains unmotivated to change, the authors
recommend services be discontinued (see also, Criteria for
Entrance and Dismissal section).

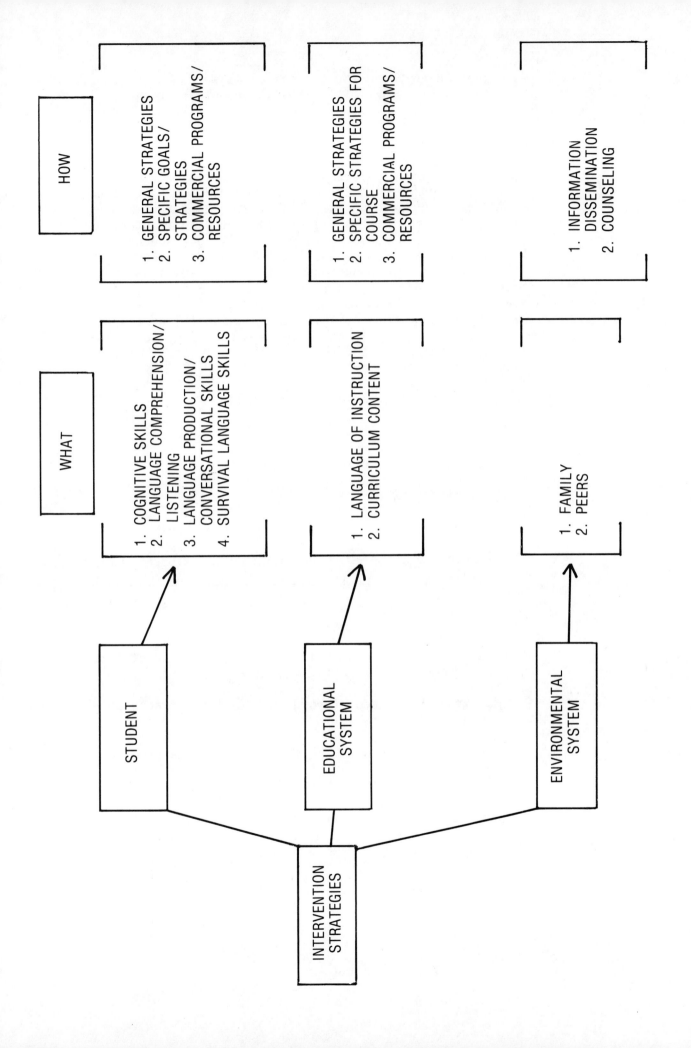

HOW

1. GENERAL STRATEGIES
2. SPECIFIC GOALS/
   STRATEGIES
3. COMMERCIAL PROGRAMS/
   RESOURCES

1. GENERAL STRATEGIES
2. SPECIFIC STRATEGIES FOR
   COURSE
3. COMMERCIAL PROGRAMS/
   RESOURCES

1. INFORMATION
   DISSEMINATION
2. COUNSELING

WHAT

1. COGNITIVE SKILLS
2. LANGUAGE COMPREHENSION/
   LISTENING
3. LANGUAGE PRODUCTION/
   CONVERSATIONAL SKILLS
4. SURVIVAL LANGUAGE SKILLS

1. LANGUAGE OF INSTRUCTION
2. CURRICULUM CONTENT

1. FAMILY
2. PEERS

STUDENT

EDUCATIONAL
SYSTEM

ENVIRONMENTAL
SYSTEM

INTERVENTION
STRATEGIES

We cannot do anything _for_ someone else; we can only provide the setting that will allow someone to help him or
herself.

C. <u>Be Prepared to Counsel</u>

The educator who provides services to adolescents with
language disorders can anticipate counseling many of them,
in addition to teaching specific strategies for communication skills. Simon (1981) has commented that intervention with certain adolescents may involve 50% speech-
language work and 50% counseling. Educators would be
well-advised to use behaviors during their sessions that
communicate understanding to teen-agers. Baggett (1969),
studying youth from rural environments, high socio-economic
communities, and correctional schools, identified the
first six behaviors listed below as most likely to communicate understanding and the last six as least likely to
communicate understanding:

1. Suggesting ways to solve the problem

2. Taking time to sit down and talk

3. Spending time to discuss the problem

4. Listening to what the student has to say

5. Asking the student questions about the problem

6. Sticking to the problem about which the student wants
   to talk _____

7. Jumping to conclusions before the student finishes
   giving the facts

8. Changing the topic immediately after the student introduces concern

9. Hurrying the student through the telling of an experience

10. Avoiding talking with the student about the problem

11. Sitting there "like a bump on a log"

12. Looking at something else while the student is talking

D. Adjust to the Social-Cognitive Development of Students

As previously indicated in the manual, adolescence is a time of major transition in social-cognitive skills. As a group, students in Grades 7-9 are intellectually and socially different from older adolescents in Grades 10-12. This has implications for how we intervene. Major implications are outlined by Ritter (1981):

1. Design curricula which stimulates development toward formal operational thinking rather than assuming students have already reached that period. Most junior and senior high school students have not yet attained formal operational thought; others are inexperienced in this mode of thinking; and yet others fail to apply it to their communicative behavior.

2. Design intervention activities emphasize "doing" communication in an instrumental sense since most students are at a concrete operational level. Introducing formal operational aspects such as persuasive tactics are not usually productive for opening activities.

3. Design intervention to involve a group process rather than individual work. Group activities allow adolescents to interact and learn from one another, a consistent theme that is emphasized in cognitive developmental literature. Discussion is particularly appropriate.

4. Design activities that are sensitive to the peer pressure felt during adolescence. Peer influence and conformity reach greatest intensity by ages eleven to thirteen and decline slowly thereafter. Classes emphasizing speech are "risky" for adolescents because of their public nature. For example, a student who is required to "pick something that interests you to talk about" may be devastated to discover that the peer group finds the topic choice peculiar.

5. Design activities that encourage the students to become increasingly responsive to each other. Early adolescents are primarily concerned with themselves and are convinced that others are also preoccupied with their appearance and behavior. The adolescent is continually constructing or reacting to an imaginary audience; this probably accounts for typical behaviors such as extreme self-consciousness, constant preening, and adolescent boorishness. In the 14 to 17 year age range, adolescents are better able to consider different perspectives and to engage in appropriate interpersonal communication behaviors based on another's needs.

141

E. Be Cognizant of Adult Learning Theory

There is a growing body of information available on the topic of adult learning (Knowles, 1973). The authors do not mean to imply that adolescents are adults, but neither are they small children. Older adolescents may be developing learning patterns that are more typical of adults than of children. Educators providing intervention services for this age group should be aware that adult learning theory does exist and that it could have ramifications for certain students on the caseload.

F. Establish Ground Rules for Intervention Sessions

The need to establish basic rules for communication occurring during intervention is addressed in the section entitled "Intervention Strategies: Language Production/ Conversational Skills." In addition to following rules that affect conversations and discussion, it is strongly recommended that speech-language pathologists establish rules of confidentiality with students particularly since counseling is sometimes necessary. Students need to feel secure that what they say and do will remain a private matter between themselves and the educator. If you sense it would be better that certain information not be shared by a student within a group session, arrange a private meeting time with the individual student. Few events cause more mistrust in you and in the services provided than a breech in confidentiality.

III. SUMMARY

General intervention principles include special considerations necessary for work with the adolescent population. The intervention process for older students has no hidden agenda; students play an active part in planning their program. Their rapidly changing social-cognitive development needs to be constantly kept in mind by educators if intervention is to succeed.

IV. ACTIVITIES

A. List any additional general principles under which you operate during the intervention process with adolescents.

   1.

   2.

   3.

B. List characteristics of adult learners and indicate which ones, if any, are held by your language disordered students.

   1.

   2.

   3.

INTERVENTION STRATEGIES: COGNITIVE SKILLS

I. **INTRODUCTION**

A growing number of studies support the idea that adolescents can successfully be taught thinking skills (Feuerstein, 1980; Lipman & Sharp, 1974). This section is designed to present, first, what to teach the adolescent who is having difficulty with thinking skills; and second, how to teach cognitive skills.

II. **WHAT TO TEACH**

Adequate processing at levels of input, elaboration, and output are goals for students with deficits in cognition. Specific behaviors within each of these areas have been cited in the "What to Assess" section of Cognitive Skills. Activities to enhance many of these skills are included in the next section III B.

III. **HOW TO TEACH**

This section is divided into three areas: General Strategies Specific Strategies, and Commercially Available Programs and/ or Resources that may be used to teach a variety of thinking skills/problem solving methods.

    A. **General Strategies for Teaching Problem Solving/Thinking Skills**

        1. **Instrumental Enrichment** (Feuerstein, 1980): This instructional sequence has much to offer adolescents with language disorders. The following concepts are most helpful:

            a. Mediation of cognitive structures can occur at <u>any</u> age, thus making it possible to learn continuously. Students with cognitive deficiencies need an adult to anchor experiences for them in time, space, and affect. For example, a direction should include, explicitly or implicitly, when and where a task is to be accomplished, and why it has been assigned. Tone of voice, nonverbal cues and selection of words should convey affect.

            b. Bridging the thinking strategies applied in one problem solving situation to similar situations is crucial.

144

i. Maxi-bridging (content bridging) relates problems in specific subject areas.

ii. Mini-bridging relates problems in "real life."

c. Group discussion is mandatory for developing problem solving/thinking skills. Suggestions for facilitating discussion follow:

   i. Introduction: Plan time to discuss the problem presented. Have the student identify what the problem is as well as suggest possible strategies for solution.

   Questions from the instructor would include:

   -- What information have you been given?

   -- Does anything look familiar to you? If so, what?

   -- What information do we need to find?

   -- What is the problem?

   -- How do you think we're going to solve it?

   ii. Summary: Plan time to summarize the strategies used to solve a particular problem and to bridge those strategies to other situations.

   Questions could include:

   -- What did you think about to solve this problem?

   -- When else would you use that strategy (in a particular subject or in your day-to-day living)?

   -- Did you have to switch strategies? When? Why?

   iii. Process: Plan time to explore the student's thinking process, not just the final product. Ask at least as much, or more, about the student's correct answers as about the incorrect ones.

Questions could include:

--How did you figure that out?

--What could be another answer?

--What would be the best (most relevant) answer? Why?

d. Cognitive dissonance or disequilibrium is a necessary ingredient for the development of thinking skills. If students are not "uncomfortable" at times, there is no motivation for change. Do not rescue; allow them to struggle to find the solution.

2. Thinking: Strategies and Methods (Alley and Deshler, 1979) This chapter from Alley and Deshler's book Teaching the Learning Disabled Adolescent: Strategies and Methods is a thorough presentation of techniques for teaching general thinking behaviors and problem solving strategies as derived from numerous educational sources. It emphasizes the importance of the student's ability to:

a. Demonstrate general thinking behaviors as indicated by the following:

i. Students should observe and describe objects and events (e.g., "What do you notice here?")

ii. Students should develop concepts (e.g., "How would you define __x__?")

iii. Students should compare and contrast objects and events (e.g., "How is that different (same as)....?")

iv. Students should hypothesize (e.g., "What do you think causes....?")

v. Students should generalize (e.g., "When else would this occur?")

vi. Students should predict outcomes (e.g., "What would happen if....?"

vii. Students should explain an event or relationship (e.g., "What makes you think that would happen?")

146

viii. Students should offer alternatives to a problem or situation (e.g., "Can someone give me a different idea of what would happen?")

b. Demonstrate problem solving skills

    i. Students should identify and define the problem in his/her own words.

    ii. Students should analyze the problem, breaking it down into smaller steps.

    iii. Students should state the desired outcome of the problem.

    iv. Students should propose alternatives to solving the problem.

    v. Students should analyze the alternatives that he/she has generated.

    vi. Students should select the best solution from the alternatives listed.

    vii. Students should implement that solution, or describe the implementation.

    viii. Students should evaluate the solution implemented.

3. Basic Skills Guidelines for thinking/problem solving are becoming available from more and more states. For example, Vermont's State Board of Education (January, 1979) set minimum reasoning skills and added them to high school graduation requirements effective with the Class of 1983. The following skills are emphasized:

a. Have the student observe and report data from an experience.

b. Have the student identify the problem or issue presented in an experience.

c. Have the student suggest possible causes of a problem.

d. Have the student suggest some solutions to a problem.

e. Have the student predict consequences of problem solutions.

f. Have the student identify similarities and differences between items.

g. Have the student put items into groups designated
by others.

h. Have the student put items into his/her own
groups and explain the criteria used.

i. Have the student put items into serial order.

j. Have the student distinguish between statements
of fact and statements of opinion.

k. Given a dilemma situation, have the student take
at least two positions and give reasons for each.

l. From a chart, graph, table, map, or list of facts,
have the student state a summary or conclusion
based on the data.

m. From a list of data and several possible conclusions, have the student identify those conclusions
which could be validly drawn from the data.

n. Have the student gather at least three different
sources of data for a given topic.

o. Have the student select and organize data on a
given topic into a meaningful report.

You may wish to check with your state to see what is
currently being suggested with regard to curriculum
goals in the area of thinking. A number of states are
publishing guides for use by secondary school personnel.
Some of their general strategies may be applicable to
adolescents with language disorders.

B. Specific Strategies for Teaching Problem Solving/Thinking
Skills

The following strategies from the work of Feuerstein (1980)
can be used when there are deficits at the input, elaborational, and output levels.

1. Goals and Activities to Demonstrate Adequate Cognitive
Skills at the Input Level

a. Improve the collection of clear and complete information by having the student use his/her senses
(e.g., telling what is seen, heard, felt, tasted,
etc.).

148

b. Improve the student's use of a system or plan so important information is not missed. Appropriate activities would include:

   i. Have the student organize data into a chart or table.

   ii. Have the student use systematic search to find a small item mixed with an assortment of other objects.

c. Improve the student's use of labels so that he/she can remember experiences more clearly and talk about them more efficiently. Whenever nonspecific words appear, require that the student supply the appropriate name or label. Appropriate activities would include:

   i. Produce sentences containing nonspecific words. Have the students identify the nonspecific word and provide a specific label that might be appropriate (e.g., they're going trick or treating with me again this Halloween). The student would need to identify the nonspecific word (they're) and supply a reasonable substitute.

   ii. Have students participate in barrier games. Before the session, ask one of the students to use a large number of nonspecific words such as "Whatchamacallit," "Things," and "Stuff." Observe whether the other students can identify these words and ask appropriate questions to gain more specific labels.

d. Improve the student's description of events and objects (i.e., where and when they occur).

e. Improve conservation of constancies by having the student decide what characteristics of an object or event always stay the same. Appropriate activities would include:

   i. Have the student identify a specific geographical shape within several collages, keeping its size and shape constant but varying its orientation.

   ii. Have the student discuss which characteristics of the school stay the same from year to year and which change each year as different groups of students attend that school.

149

f. Improve organization of gathered information by having the student consider more than one source of information at a time. Appropriate activities would include:

 i. Have the student prioritize the kind of candy bar to buy, given information on its price, weight of the bar itself, and nutritional information. Personal preferences may also be considered.

 ii. Have the student collect information on a job field that is of personal interest. Several resources need to be used. Read the information to the student or tape-record it, if necessary. From this information, have the student organize strengths and weaknesses of the job field, characteristics one needed to enter the field and ways to get training in the field.

g. Improve the student's precision and accuracy of language production. Appropriate activities would include:

 i. Have the student participate in barrier games, particularly those requiring specific descriptions of objects or locations. For example, given the same map, have one student describe to the other how to get from location A to location B.

 ii. Have the student describe a person not in the room so that other students could identify the person being described.

 iii. Have the student simulate leaving a message about a meeting with someone so that there would be no question about who the meeting was for, what it was about, where and when it was taking place.

2. Goals and Activities to Demonstrate Adequate Cognitive Skills at the Elaborational Level

a. Improve problem identification by having the student define what the problem is, what he/she is being asked to do, what must be figured out. Appropriate activities would include:

 i. Present a printed page from a workbook minus any written instructions. Have the student explore the possible problem to be solved on the page.

150

ii. Have the student discuss what the problem is in a given situation (e.g., Bill
calls to ask you to go to the show tonight,
but you've already told Wendy you'll go
with her).

b. Improve problem solving abilities by having the
student decide what is relevant and what is irrelevant information. Appropriate activities would
include:

i. Have the student read through the instructions to a worksheet. Prior to the session,
unnecessary information has been added to
the instructions. Have the student identify
what information is irrelevant.

ii. Have the student decide what information
is irrelevant to solving a problem. For
example, add this information to the example
cited above: "Bill is calling to ask you to
the show tonight, but you've already told
Wendy you'll go with her. She is worried
about her babysitting job the next day because she has never cared for an infant before."

c. Improve problem solving by having the student form
a good picture in his/her mind of what must be
done. Appropriate activities would include:

i. Have the student describe what he/she
is thinking about while solving a problem,
particularly one that would require visuali-
zation (e.g., taking the perspective of
another person)

ii. Have the student construct a part into a
whole after being shown the final product,
without the opportunity to refer back to
it.

d. Improve problem solving by having the student make
a plan that includes steps needed to reach a solution. Appropriate activities would include:

i. Have the student list the steps that he/
she went through to reach a solution. This
plan may be written by students or verbally
reported and recorded by the adult present.

ii. Present a plan that is missing some
steps and have the student identify what
is excluded. For example, the plan is to
go on a backpacking trip. The plan presented to the student includes provisions
for food, bedding, and appropriate clothing.
However, it has excluded provisions for
maps, water-liquids, or any things that
might have to be done before leaving such
as paying bills, finding someone to care
for the dog, and taking in the mail.

e. Improve problem solving by having the student
remember the various pieces of information needed
to solve the problem. Appropriate activities
would include:

i. Give the student a list of errands to run
in the community. Some would take little
time; others would take longer and necessi-
tate conforming to business hours. The student would be asked to plan the most efficient manner of performing the errands, keeping in mind the location of the stop and the
time needed.

ii. Present a number of geometrical forms
varying in size and number. Ask the student
to draw a picture next to each form(s) so
that shape and number are different, but the
size is always the same. In order to do
this task, the student needs to remember the
rules throughout the variety of forms.

f. Improve problem solving by having the student
look for the relationship among separate objects,
events, and experiences. Appropriate activities
would include:

i. Have the student bridge a strategy in one
thinking situation to that used in another.
(For example, fading out of cues is common
when learning a new activity. After encoun-
tering a task, when cues have faded, ask the
student what else he/she has learned through
the process of gradually fading cues.)

ii. Have the student describe the relationship between or among objects that differ
in many attributes, but share at least one
common quality. For example, a door and a
box share 90° angles.

g. Improve comparisons of objects and experiences by having the student see similarities and differences. Appropriate activities would include:

   i. Have the student describe how any two words presented are alike and how they are different. (For example, given the words "flour" and "water," what is something that they share, and what is something that is different about them?)

   ii. Have the student discuss words like "similar," "same," "identical," etc. Why is it necessary for us to have so many words that seem to describe essentially the same phenomena?

h. Improve problem solving by having the student categorize new objects. Appropriate activities would include:

   i. Have the student supply a category heading when given a list of words in writing or verbally.

   ii. After the above task, have the student supply category words above and below the ones given within their respective hierarchies (e.g., if the word "fruit" was supplied above, the additional category words might be "food" and "citrus").

i. Improve problem solving by having the student think about different possibilities, using hypothetical thinking to figure out what would happen if he/she were to choose another option. Appropriate activities would include:

   i. Have the student identify when he/she switches strategies to solve a problem. Describe the change. (For example, my strategy for finishing my homework was to do it Sunday night, but when I found out my grandmother was coming, I switched my plans to Saturday night.)

   ii. Have the student describe why it was necessary to switch strategies. (For example, it might be to save time, energy, or money, or to cope with interruption.)

j. Improve problem solving by having the student use logic to prove solutions and to defend opinions.

   i. Have the student answer the question, "How did you get that answer?" Push for use of logical rationale.

   ii. Have the student answer questions such as "What makes you feel/believe that?", especially as it refers to opinions that they hold rather than to facts. (For example, "Why do you feel that pizza is the best fast food available?")

3. Goals and Activities for Demonstration of Adequate Cognitive Skills at the Output Level

   a. Improve problem solving by having the student use clear and concise language in order to ensure that the answer is clear. Appropriate activities would include:

      i. Have the student participate in barrier games as previously described.

      ii. Present questions with multiple choice answers and have the student identify on a continuum what answers are the clearest and what answers are the least clear.

   b. Improve problem solving by having the student think the answer through instead of immediately trying to answer and making a mistake (i.e., trial and error). Appropriate activities would include:

      i. Have the student discuss the idea that "thinking takes time." How does it feel to be under pressure to produce an answer in a short amount of time? Why do people on television quiz shows fail to answer questions that appear simple to you and me?

      ii. Discuss when trial and error is a desirable strategy for solving a problem. In what situations might it be used?

   c. Improve problem solving by having the student restrain impulsive behavior, doing things which he/she will be sorry for later. Appropriate activities would include:

i. Have the student discuss why it is important to restrain impulsive behavior. What
can be gained by learning to control behavior?

ii. Have the student develop comprehension
and production of the word "impulsive."
Apply the word to situations in which the
student is using impulsive behavior.

d. Improve problem solving by having the student
avoid panic or frustration when he/she cannot answer a question even though the answer is known.
The student may leave the question for a while,
then return to it and use a strategy to help find
the answer.

C. Commercially Available Programs/Resources

1. Problem Solving: Using Your Head Creatively (Human
Relations Media, 1978) is a very good overview-
introduction to problem solving. Made up of four
filmstrips and cassettes, it outlines basic strategies for any problem solving situation including
those in human relationships.

2. Let's Look at Logic (Guidance Associates, 1977) contains filmstrips, cassettes, and logic cards. The
cards may be of particular use to the speech-language
pathologist. Example cards include these items:

a. Decide whether or not this reasoning is correct:
"You really should not order your hamburger well
done since good hamburgers are rare these days."

b. Decide whether or not this reasoning is correct:
"Sandra did not get good grades in science. If
she were a boy, she would have gotten good grades."

c. The highest card in a sequence gives the following problem: "All P's are Q's. Some Y's are Q's.
Problem: Are some P's Y's?"

3. Think Lab (Weber, 1974) is designed to be used from
adolescence through adulthood. It includes these
levels of thinking:

a. Object manipulation, which involves the collection
of specific data

b. Perception, which extrapolates from data provided

c. Creative insight

d. Perception of image patterns/analysis of structure

e. Logical analysis, which includes hypothesis test-
    ing and operations planning

The emphasis may be on thinking skills that are on a
higher level than many adolescents with language disorders could profit from without a more basic, preceding curriculum.

4. Successful Problem Solving Techniques (Greenes, 1977)
    is a straightforward approach to problem solving.
    The text provides a general strategy for problem solv-
    ing as well as two chapters of worksheets that can be
    reproduced for students. Designed for Grades 6-12,
    the speech-language pathologist could "pick and choose"
    specific problems.

    Many of the problems are math-oriented. Sample prob-
    lems are:

    a. How many different ways can you make change for
        a 50-cent piece without using pennies?

    b. I saw a cat in the middle, two cats in front of
        a cat, and two cats behind a cat. What is the
        smallest number of cats I could have seen?

    c. Five friends were sitting on one side of a table
        in a cafeteria. Bill sat next to Sally, Joe sat
        next to Ed, Ruth sat in the third seat from
        Sally, and Bill sat in the third seat from Joe.
        Who sat on the other side of Ed?

5. Cognitive Challenge Cards (Ross, 1978) are based on
    Bloom's taxonomy, and could be quite useful to the
    professional teaching problem solving skills. Prob-
    lems are presented that require analysis of attributes,
    determination of relevant versus irrelevant informa-
    tion, and use of questioning strategies as well as
    other skills.

6. Attribute Games: Problem Solving and Reasoning Skills
    Development (Marshall, 1971) provides a set of 60
    small blocks consisting of five shapes, three colors,
    two sizes, and two thicknesses. The forms are excel-
    lent for grouping sets, illustrating intersections and
    unions of sets and demonstrating Venn diagrams. Games
    such as the following are also suggested:

a. Two Dimensional Game: Establish a vertical row of forms that vary by one attribute and a horizontal row of forms that vary by two attributes. Have students systematically add additional forms conforming to the rules established.

b. Matrix Game: A matrix outline is used (e.g., 7 x 7 grid, or 49 spaces). Attribute blocks are placed at each corner and players determine how many attributes must be varied by each adjacent form. Players take turns filling in the matrix. The game is varied by pre-positioning certain forms at random locations on the grid.

7. Book of Think (or How to Solve a Problem Twice Your Size) (Burns,1976) can be used at least through junior high school and possibly into senior high school. Although short on an overall strategy approach, the book does offer many opportunities for problem solving and for developing awareness of thinking processes. It also emphasizes the "smartness" of asking questions. Consider these examples:

a. How many ways can you turn a glass of water upside down without spilling the water? (Problem Solving)

b. True or False: A record on a record player turns in a clockwise direction? (Developing Awareness)

c. Imagine you are a TV interviewer. You are interviewing a famous athlete who was forced to stop playing because of a broken leg. You have time to ask only three questions. What three questions would you ask?

The Book of Think is in the Brown Paper School series by Little, Brown, and Company. Other books would also be appropriate (e.g., This Book Is About Time).

8. Harry Stottlemeier's Discovery (Institute for the Advancement of Philosophy for Children, 1977) introduces logic and philosophical concepts through an entertaining novel. Through use of a discussion format, the following objectives are pursued:

a. The improvement of the student's reasoning and ability to draw inferences

b. The development of the student's creativity, spontaneity, and imaginative thinking

c. The personal development of the student through the increased confidence and maturity that results from challenging the thought processes

d. The development of attitudes that promote logical thought through discovery (e.g., discovery of alternatives, discovery of the feasibility of giving reasons for beliefs)

9. Instrumental Enrichment (Feuerstein, 1980) Levels I and II provide an excellent comprehensive intervention curriculum that addresses all cognitive deficits. The following instruments (units) are included in the curriculum:

a. "Organization of Dots" has as its objective "to teach and provide specific practice in the projection of virtual relationships through tasks that require the student to identify and outline given figures within a cloud of dots." During work in this instrument, the following types of questions are asked:

   i. What else can we organize besides dots?

   ii. Why do we organize?

   iii. What are some of the principles (the rules) that will help us to organize?

b. "Orientation in Space I" has as its objective "to provide a stable, although relative, system of reference by which to describe spatial relationships and to produce a direct attack on the limited use of articulated, differentiated, representational space." This instrument deals specifically with the concepts of left-right and front-back.

c. "Comparisons" has a number of objectives. The instrument focuses on increasing and enriching the repertoire of attributes by which stimuli can be compared. It also attempts to turn the act of comparison into an automatic activity so that students spontaneously perceive and describe relationships among objects, events, and ideas with regard to their similarities and differences.

d. "Analytic Perception" is designed to teach strategies for synthesizing parts into a whole according to the needs of a given moment. The instrument also addresses the division of a whole into its parts in accordance with specific goals.

158

e. "Categorization" is designed to have a student organize data into categories and can also be called "Classification." The student groups objects or events according to underlying principles and subsumes them into appropriate sets.

f. "Family Relations" emphasizes relationships experienced by the student in daily living. The instrument examines not only relationships among individuals in extended families, but relationships in other systems (e.g., political, academic).

g. "Temporal Relations" addresses the student's perception of time and his/her capacity to register, process, and order temporal relationships.

h. "Numerical Progressions" focuses on the search for rules and laws that form the basis for the relationship among events.

i. "Instructions" has as its objective not only the following of directions, both explicit and implicit, but the ability to encode instruction for someone else.

j. "Illustrations" offers the student the opportunity to apply the thinking he/she has learned in all other instruments. A problem from the "Illustrations" instrument can be presented whenever the need arises. Each problem is designed to produce in a student an awareness of the existence of that problem which leads to a disruption of equilibrium and a search for a solution. "Illustrations" revolves around a humorous or absurd situation.

10. Basic Thinking Skills (Harnadek, 1977) There are eleven booklets in this series. The purpose of each booklet is to sharpen thinking skills using a class discussion format. Individual students' written responses may also be used as the format. In many cases, there is more than one acceptable answer. Some of the booklets within the series include "Analogies," "Antonyms and Synonyms," "What Would You Do? and True to Life or Fantasy?"

11. Mind Benders: Deductive Thinking Skills (Harnadek, 1978) There are seven booklets or ditto masters in this series. The purpose of the series is to force students to organize sets of data to reach logical conclusions by using deductive reasoning. There are three levels to Mind Benders -- easy, medium, and difficult. The more advanced booklets require extensive charting of data and may not be the most appropriate for students with severe language disorders.

The easiest booklet begins with a problem in transitive relationships (e.g., "Edmund, Ida, Joanne, and Tony are two sets of twins. Tony is a month younger than Edmund. Joanne is a month older than Ida. Which pair is the younger set of twins?").

12. Critical Thinking (Harnadek, 1976) The material in Critical Thinking is aimed primarily at and above the junior high school level although the reading level is at about the fifth or sixth grade. The problems are designed to provoke class discussion. The author firmly states her belief that a student learns how to think critically not by being told how to do it, but by doing it. The book contains over 1000 problems and questions and educators are urged to choose those which they think will appeal to their particular groups and to eliminate those whose interest level they think might be above or below the age level of the group. The author further encourages users of the book to question students regarding their reasons for answers.

13. Classification and Organization Skills - Developmental (Curriculum Associates, Inc., 1981) Thirty-two activities are arranged in sequential order beginning with tasks such as sorting (categorizing) words, and sorting by "who, what, where, when," progressing through alphabetizing, sequencing sentences, and paragraphs, selecting main ideas and sorting for details, and ending with organizing and completing an outline. Information presented visually could easily be presented verbally to keep reading requirements at a minimal level.

14. Thinkerthings: A Student-Generated Approach to Language Experience (Miller and Judd, 1975) Skills are emphasized in four main areas:

-- Comprehension

-- Research skills

-- Structural analysis

-- Word analysis

Specific activities include:

-- Classifying

-- Defining

-- Inferential thinking

160

-- Sequencing

-- Using prefixes and suffixes

-- Using antonyms - homonyms - synonyms

Thinkerthings is recommended for students in Grades
4-8. Many of the activities could be adapted for use
beyond eighth grade, although the illustrations in
the book are not appropriate for older students.

15. Choose Your Own Adventure Series (Bantam Books, 1981)
Two levels of this series are now available. The
high-interest stories force a choice of action after
every page or two. The skilled pathologist can present these stories orally (to eliminate the need for
reading skills) and ask relevant questions that
address basic problem solving and thinking skills.

16. Computer Programs are plentiful and can be used in a
similar manner to the "Choose Your Own Adventure"
series. For example, a computer program such as
"Oregon Trail" (Minnesota Educational Computer Con-
sortium, 1980) engages the student in a hypothetical
trek westward in the 1800's and forces him/her to
make choices regarding the number of horses or oxen
to buy, the amount of ammunition to buy, whether to
hunt on the way or to buy food, and so forth. Having
the student verbalize his/her reasoning while running
the computer program can mesh intimately with teaching thinking skills/problem solving behavior.

Virtually all computer "games" have underlying strategies that can be discussed with students. We have
only touched the tip of computer-assisted instruction.
Prepare for dramatic adjustments in the next few
years as software becomes more and more available.

IV. SUMMARY

This section presents information on the importance of teaching cognitive skills, what to teach, and how to teach it. In
the discussion of how to teach the student, the authors present general strategies, specific strategies for selected
tasks, and available commercial programs and resources.

V. ACTIVITIES

A. Select one student currently on your caseload and list
   in order of priority the major cognitive goals for this
   student.

   1.

   2.

   3.

   4.

   5.

B. With the same student in mind, list which general cognitive strategies he/she needs to learn. What are some
   additional activities for teaching them?

   General Strategies   Activities

   1.   1.

   2.   2.

   3.   3.

   4.   4.

C. With the same student in mind, list what specific cognitive strategies need to be taught. What are some additional activities for teaching them?

<u>Specific Strategies</u>   <u>Activities</u>

1.   1.

2.   2.

3.   3.

4.   4.

D. With the same student in mind, list appropriate commercial programs/resources. What elements of these programs/resources are best suited for teaching this student? What elements are least important?

1.

2.

3.

4.

INTERVENTION STRATEGIES: LANGUAGE COMPREHENSION/LISTENING

I. INTRODUCTION

As stated within the assessment section, listening is the
most important of the basic skills for success in the educational environment. This section is designed to first present
what to teach the adolescent who is having difficulty in the
area of listening and, second, how to teach listening.

II. WHAT TO TEACH

Adequate auditory comprehension of linguistic processing skills,
informational listening skills, and/or critical listening
skills are goals for students with deficits. Specific behaviors
within each of these areas have been cited in the "What to
Assess" section of listening. Activities to enhance many of
these skills are included in the next section, III B.

III. HOW TO TEACH

This section is divided into three areas: General Strategies including "Listening in the Classroom" that might be used across
subject areas; Specific Strategies for selected listening
tasks; and Commercially Available Programs and/or Resources
that may be used to teach the various types of listening.

A. General Strategies for Teaching Language Comprehension/
    Listening

    1. Enhancing Classroom Listening Skills - An Eclectic
        Pragmatic Approach

        Although the junior/senior high school student en-
        gages in various types of listening situations, one
        of the most critical for academic success is class-
        room listening. This approach is designed to enhance
        listening skills across all subject content areas and
        is derived from a variety of sources, particularly
        Alley and Deshler (1979). This approach divides the
        task into three levels: Pre-Listening, Listening,
        and Post-Listening.

        a. Pre-Listening Strategies - Using a problem solving
            approach, encourage student to:

            i. Be mentally prepared to listen.

                (a) Avoid incorrect listening habits.

164

(b) Listen actively by mentally asking questions about the material being presented.

(c) Determine the teacher's lecture style ahead of time.

(d) Review notes and materials from previous classes.

(e) Read materials related to today's class.

(f) Relate lecture topic to other topics.

(g) Develop the necessary vocabulary words that will be used in the upcoming lecture.

ii. Be physically prepared to listen.

(a) Sit near the front of the class.

(b) Bring appropriate materials to class by developing a brief checklist of materials for each class on a 3" x 5" card and keep them in your pocket or purse.

b. Listening Strategies - Within the listening situation itself, encourage the student to:

i. Listen for verbal and nonverbal cues.

(a) Using videotaped lectures, teach the student to recognize and understand frequently used verbal organizational cues such as "in summary," "as a result," "a key point," "the topic for today will be discussed under three areas." In addition, remind the student that verbal cues include vocal inflection, pause, rate, and repetition of information for emphasis.

(b) Teach the student to recognize and understand nonverbal cues such as eye contact, gestures, body position, and facial expressions to add information.

ii. Listen for main and supporting ideas.

(a) Have the student suggest titles for short paragraphs.

  (b) Tell a short story and have students summarize it in one sentence.

  (c) Have students listen to a lecture on videotape and identify the main ideas.

 iii. Question for clarification.

  (a) Students should be taught when to ask questions (e.g., during a pause or between discussion points).

  (b) Students should be taught how to ask questions (e.g., in a pleasant, polite tone of voice).

  (c) Students should be taught what type of questions obtain what type of information (e.g., why questions yield causal explanations).

 iv. Seek and use feedback.

  (a) Students should be taught how nonverbal communication can indicate to the teacher that they need clarification (e.g., a puzzled look, a wrinkled brow, or a scowl).

  (b) Students should learn to "read" the other listeners (e.g., Are they bored?).

  (c) Students should learn to use feedback both verbally and nonverbally as a way of informing the teacher of how effectively the message is coming through.

 v. Apply memory strategies.

The three memory strategies that might be applied are:

  (a) Rehearsal strategy (repeating to one-self information just heard to promote its retention)

  (b) Visual imagery of material to retain information

  (c) Clustering and coding information (used to increase listening effectiveness and recall-association)

vi. Take notes to facilitate listening.

    (a) Students should determine if notes will be helpful.

    (b) Students should decide on the most effective way to take notes (i.e., complete outline, partial outline, or key words).

    (c) Students should learn to take clear and brief notes.

    (d) Students should appropriately use listening guides supplied by the teacher.

c. Post-Listening Strategies

  i. These review strategies consist of the following:

    (a) Students should review their notes after class and add information that they did not have an opportunity to record in class.

    (b) Students should question themselves to confirm understanding of the information.

    (c) Students should draw a set of summary statements or conclusions.

  ii. Students should skim their notes before the next class. Skimming concludes post-listening strategies and acts as a pre-listening activity.

We have found this pre-listening, listening, and post-listening strategy approach to be most successful in facilitating classroom listening skills for junior/ senior high students.

2. Basic Skills Guidelines for listening are becoming available from various states. For example, Vermont's State Board of Education (March, 1977) set minimum listening skills requirements for high school graduation effective with the Class of 1983. The following skills are emphasized:

a. Have the student listen to three-step oral directions once and follow them with 100% accuracy.

b. Have the student listen to a story and then re-
    tell the significant events sequentially, either
    orally or in written form.

c. Have the student listen to an oral presentation
    and then summarize the essential details of the
    presentation.

You should check to see if your state has adopted
basic competencies in listening required for graduation from high school. Such basic competencies may
provide guidelines for general strategies developed
during intervention.

B. Specific Strategies for Teaching Listening Skills

1. Goals and Activities for Auditory Comprehension of
    Linguistic Processing Skills

    a. Improve comprehension of morphological features

        i.   Improve comprehension of noun plurals and
             noun-verb agreement by using a multiple
             choice cloze procedure (e.g., "Mary takes
             one (book/books) to school." "The boy
             (play/plays) baseball.").

        ii. Improve comprehension of suffixes and pre-
             fixes by having the student identify and
             learn the meaning of a variety of root
             words, prefixes, and suffixes. Also, use
             a segmentation activity where the student
             divides words into their smallest meaning-
             ful units and discuss the meaning of the
             suffix or prefix.

        iii. Improve comprehension of verb tenses with
             activities that allow the student to dif-
             ferentiate between past, present, and future
             by using words such as yesterday, today, and
             tomorrow as cues to the appropriate verb
             tense. Discuss verb tenses in terms of the
             phonological rules which condition the use
             of a specific suffix.

        iv. Improve comprehension of comparatives and
             superlatives by first establishing the cog-
             nitive base for these forms of adjectives
             (size, length, weight, or quality) and then
             use multiple choice cloze procedures.

    b. Improve comprehension of syntactic features

168

i. Improve comprehension of the different types of sentences (declarative, interrogative, imperative, negative, passive) by having the student identify sentences from nonsentences and identify the various types of sentences and explain the meaning of each.

ii. Improve comprehension of conjoined and embedded sentences by first establishing that the student has the cognitive base for the various conjunctives and can identify the component dependent and independent clauses. Also, the student should understand the functional use (purpose) of independent and dependent clauses and conjunctives. Activities can include using multiple choice cloze procedures.

c. Improve comprehension of semantic features

i. Improve comprehension of antonyms, synonyms, and homonyms by progressing from using concrete words frequently to using more abstract ones less frequently. Provide activities for the student that teach words in pairs (e.g., big-little, big-large, and sail-sale). Also, multiple choice cloze procedures and spontaneous cloze procedures can be used to enhance sentence comprehension.

ii. Improve comprehension of multiple meaning of words by introducing the various meanings of a word such as "run." Use the word in a sentence and have the student provide the meaning based on the context.

2. Goals and Activities for Informational Listening

a. Improve informational listening by having the students identify, describe, and analyze situations in which they would prefer not to listen. Also, have the student describe situations in which poor listening habits could cause problems.

b. Improve informational listening by having the student listen in spite of auditory and/or visual distractions (e.g., listen while a radio is playing or when sitting next to a window where activity is going on outside).

c. Improve comprehension by having the student detect the main idea of a paragraph presented orally. Appropriate activities would include:

i. Give the student the definition of a main idea.

ii. Have the student find the main idea of a paragraph. Read short paragraphs to the student, then have him/her choose the main idea from a multiple-choice activity. Increase the difficulty of the task through increasing the length of the paragraphs and requiring students to explain in their own words the purpose of the paragraph.

iii. Have the student find the main idea by listening to an audiotape of a lecture presentation or one of their teacher's paragraphs, and picking out main ideas.

iv. Have the student listen to announcements, short articles from the newspaper, history articles, stories of inventions or inventors, TV commentaries, or the news. Have the student identify the why, who, what, where, and when of the article or story. The student must learn to answer these WH questions about articles and stories in order to be more informed.

d. Improve comprehension by having the student discriminate, through listening, between important ideas and extra details. An appropriate activity might involve having the student listen to a story and then label given sentences as important ideas or extra details.

e. Improve comprehension by having the student outline a short paragraph after (or while) listening to it. An appropriate activity would be to have the clinician read a short informative paragraph to the student, who is provided with a skeleton outline giving only the main topic lines. The student must fill in the details as the paragraph is read.

f. Improve comprehension by having the student take effective notes from a variety of lectures. An appropriate activity would be to have the student tape-record the lecture and take notes on a five-minute segment, then analyze the note taking methods.

g. Improve comprehension to recall a series of events or objects presented auditorially. An appropriate activity would be to have the clinician read a list of names, objects, or events and to have the student recall them in the sequence given. For example, "Traveling down the road I saw a Vega, Toyota, Mercedes, and Firebird."

h. Improve comprehension to ask appropriate questions about an auditorially presented paragraph. An appropriate activity would be to read short paragraphs to the student. The paragraph will leave out an idea important to the understanding of the material, and the student must ask an appropriate question to understand the paragraph.

3. Goals and Activities for Critical Listening

a. Improve comprehension by having the student detect hasty generalizations. Appropriate activites might include:

i. Stress that the soundness of any generalization or conclusion depends on the amount of evidence that supports it (e.g., "All teen-agers are rude" cannot be said on the basis that a few may be).

ii. Have the student find examples of hasty generalizations in newspapers, magazines, on TV, and in instructors' lectures.

b. Improve comprehension by having the student recognize either-or thinking. An appropriate activity might include having the student suggest specific examples of either-or reasoning. Some possible examples are: right or wrong; good or bad; intelligent or stupid; with us or against us.

c. Improve comprehension by having the student recognize cause and effect relationships. Appropriate activities might include having the student bring in examples of faulty cause and effect thinking from every day life (e.g., superstitions and home remedies).

d. Improve comprehension to recognize and use inductive and deductive reasoning.

i. Have the student recognize and apply inductive reasoning. Appropriate activities would illustrate ways in which we reach con-

171

clusions after observing evidence (facts, examples, statistics). This is reasoning from the specific to the general.

ii. Have the student recognize and apply deductive reasoning. An appropriate activity could define deductive reasoning as that which begins with a generalization and follows logical steps to lead to a conclusion about a particular situation. This is reasoning from the general to the specific.

iii. Have the student recognize propaganda devices.

(a) The student should become aware that listeners are more vulnerable than readers. Appropriate activities include: defining propaganda as a form of persuasion that attempts to influence opinion, judgment, and action primarily through appeals to emotions rather than to intellect. Have the student keep a notebook on propaganda devices seen in newspapers or heard on the radio or TV.

(b) The student should recognize loaded words. An appropriate activity would point out the differences in feelings in the following words: "William is fat versus overweight versus husky."

Also, warn students that loaded words lead listeners to associate things that they have heard with things for which they have already developed feelings. What is the difference, for example, between crowd, mob, gang, and club?

(c) The student should recognize name calling. Appropriate activities might include compiling lists of names commonly used to attack someone ("Communist," "sissy," "Hippie", "Fascist," "punk," "moron") and select examples of name calling from newspaper editorials and political speeches.

(d) The student should recognize slogans. Activities might include stressing the fact that while they may be easily remembered, slogans over-simplify and

172

do not give any real information. Have the student compile lists of popular slogans and create slogans to popularize a product.

   (e) The student should recognize bandwagon techniques. An appropriate activity might develop an awareness of "Bandwagon Techniques" by asking students for examples such as, "Aw, Mom, why can't I stay out until 1:00 a.m.? All the other kids can."

   (f) The student should recognize testimonial techniques. Activities might include discussing testimonial devices wherein a well-known person testifies about the worth of a product, idea, or cause and explaining that testimonials can be valid if the people making the endorsement are qualified experts. Use the following checklist:

      -- Who is the speaker?

      -- What qualifies him as a reliable authority?

      -- What are his motives?

      -- Does he support his opinion with facts and reasons?

C. Commercially Available Programs/Resources

   1. Listening: Readings (Duker, 1971) This is, as the name implies, a book of readings which has several chapters on listening assessment and programming for junior/senior high students.

   2. Effective Listening (Xerox Corporation, 1967) This is a program designed initially for business people. It has in the introduction an article by Ralph Nichols and Leonard Stevens. The program is designed to enhance the listener's ability to recall main ideas and supporting details, recognize fact from opinion, etc. It uses a pre-test and a post-test format. This program might be used with secondary level students.

   3. Listening Skills Development (Eggleston and Riggs, 1982) Intermediate level. This program has a pre-test and post-test format. The auditory tapes, manual, and workbook include the following units:

a. Following simple directions

b. Decoding with context cues

c. Interpreting situational clues

d. Recognizing and recalling details

e. Recalling sequences

f. Identifying similarities

g. Drawing inferences and making generalizations

h. Identifying cause and effect

i. Interpreting main ideas

j. Following more complex directions

k. Examining sources

l. Detecting nonsense

m. Separating fact and opinion

n. Recognizing emotional language

o. Analyzing relevance of information

p. Identifying unsupported statements

q. Identifying missing elements

r. Recognizing ad Hominum response

4. Improving Aural Comprehension (Morley, 1972) This is a workbook and teachers' manual designed to increase auditory comprehension of the following:

a. Numeral relationships

b. Letters

c. Sounds

d. Abbreviations

e. Spelling and alphabetizing

f. Directions and spatial relations

g. Time and temporal sequence

h. Dates and chronological order

i.   Measurements and amounts

j.   Proportion

k.   Comparison and contrast

It also includes a unit that combines the above into what is called "getting the facts."

5. Human Communication Handbook - Volume I and II (Ruben, 1975 and 1978) These books have a series of simulation activities on all aspects of communication and ways to analyze and enhance communication skills. There are specific simulation activities in both volumes that enhance listening skills within a total communication context.

6. Radio Listening (Myers, 1979) Although radio is not the dominant entertainment medium for young people that it was prior to 1950, the advent of the transistor radio has undoubtedly made radio listening a popular pastime among teen-agers.

This article includes activities such as assigning the student to listen to three different radio personalities (e.g., sports commentator, disc jockey, newscaster) for five minutes each. Using a worksheet, the student might then respond to questions such as:

a.   Did the speaker exhibit a sense of humor? How was it communicated?

b.   Did the speaker show any kind of bias or prejudice toward anything during the time you listened? What was said that would indicate some bias? Did you find that you were biased toward the speaker either positively or negatively?

c.   Did the speaker appear knowledgeable about what he/she was doing?

d.   Was the manner of delivery phoney or natural?

The list of questions can go on. The authors found that adolescents enjoy listening to the radio for main ideas and supporting details.

7. Active Listening Activities (Faix, 1975) This article discusses ways to teach active listening as a social process. Active listening is based on both verbal and nonverbal giving and receiving of information that accords and facilitates a climate of trust and acceptance, and seeks a non-judgmental openness and patience.

Activities mentioned in this article revolve around students placing themselves in groups of two, four, or six, and interviewing each other, sharing feelings and attitudes about common experiences, and attempting to be empathetic toward what they are listening to.

8. <u>Building Listening Accountability</u> (Williams, 1974) This article advocates using role playing and simulation activities to enhance listening accountability. Additional strategies are used for building interest and motivation, increasing tolerance for conflict and ambiguity, and forming a questioning and critical attitude.

9. <u>Listening Guides</u> (Castello, 1976) Listening Guides are considered a first step toward teaching students note-taking. It assists them in listening for main points in a lecture. The student is given an outline of the key points of the lecture and space to fill in additional information. This article emphasizes that rather than teach students how to go about organizing words on paper, we must first organize these words ourselves and then tell our students what those words are.

10. <u>Old Time Radio Listening</u> (McLeod, 1979) Today's teenagers appear to be fascinated by the old time radio programs of the 1940's. They are highly motivated and interested in listening and visually fantasizing about what they hear.

   The following list of projects from McLeod (1979) suggests sundry activities students could be engaged in with Old Time Radio (OTR). These activities are suited for middle school through college level students.

   a. Design and conduct trivia quizzes modeled after Old Time Radio.

   b. Conduct a radio show based on an Old Time Radio presentation.

   c. Compare advertising techniques then and now.

   d. Compare Old Time Radio to modern radio, especially in terms of programming.

   e. Design sets of questions for shows.

   f. Find words which have changed in meaning.

11. <u>Teaching Critical Listening</u> (Tutolo, 1975) Tutolo provides a three-step program to teach critical listening skills:

STEP ONE: The students analyze advertisements as to needs the product appeals to such as:

-- <u>Self-Actualization</u> (becoming all one can be)

-- <u>Esteem needs</u> (competence, mastery, adequacy-achievement recognition)

-- <u>Love needs</u> (affection and belonging)

-- <u>Safety needs</u> (freedom from bodily illness and danger)

-- <u>Physiological needs</u> (including food, water, air, etc.)

STEP TWO: The student analyzes the ad in terms of propaganda devices such as:

-- Name calling

-- Glittering

-- Transfer

-- Testimonial

-- Card Stacking

-- Identification

-- Bandwagon

STEP THREE: The student is to draw a conclusion about whether or not to buy the product. The article includes a series of questions and a checklist designed for this activity.

12. <u>Directed Listening Activity</u> (Cunningham and Cunningham, 1976) Directed Listening consists of at least three stages: readiness; reading-recitation; and follow-up. The authors suggest specific activities within these stages.

13. Guided Listening (Cunningham and Cunningham, 1976)
    In the guided listening procedure, the teacher se-
    lects some material for the students to hear. The
    teacher may give a lecture, or play a record or tape.
    The selection should not exceed 10 minutes of total
    listening time. The teacher then proceeds through a
    nine-step process.

    The first eight steps can be completed in 50 minutes
    or less if the listening selection is 10 minutes or
    less.

14. Listening and Note-taking (DiVesta and Gray, 1972
    and 1973) These are simply experimental studies
    demonstrating the interrelationship between listen-
    ing and note-taking during lectures in order to re-
    call information later.

15. A Program to Improve Listening (N.E.A., 1964) The
    National Educational Association has listed a number
    of factors that they believe should be part of a pro-
    gram to improve listening. They are:

    a. Creating the proper listening climate

    b. Improving listening attitudes

    c. Teaching listening as a tool for learning

    d. Providing planned instruction in certain listen-
        ing skills

16. Listening In and Speaking Out (James, Whitley, and
    Bode, 1980) This is a set of audiotaped stories and
    a workbook which accompanies them. The intent of the
    program is to teach students to listen for the main
    ideas, increase their vocabulary comprehension, sum-
    marize information, retell the story, and use the
    cloze procedure to listen for specific words.

17. Reading Listening Comprehension Skills (Insel and
    Edson, 1976) This program consists of five audio-
    tape cassettes with ten individualized lessons, one
    for each of nine basic skills, plus a pre-test for
    diagnosis and a post-test for determining whether
    the behavioral objectives were accomplished. The
    students are to learn the following:

    a. Follow verbal directions

    b. Determine sequence of events

    c. Recall details

d. Predict outcomes

e. Identify main idea and details

f. Interpret main idea and details

g. Recognize cause and effect

h. Infer causation

i. Make inferences

j. Distinguish main idea from details

k. Interpret figurative speech

l. Select best title

m. Distinguish fact and opinion

IV. <u>SUMMARY</u>

This section presents information on the importance of teaching language comprehension/listening skills, what to teach, and how to teach it. In the discussion of how to teach the student, the authors present general strategies, specific strategies for selected tasks, and available commercial programs and resources.

V. ACTIVITIES

A. Select one student currently on your caseload and list in order of priority the major language comprehension/ listening goals for this student.

   1.

   2.

   3.

   4.

B. With the same student in mind, list which general language comprehension/listening strategies he/she needs to learn. What are some additional activities for teaching them?

   General Strategies   Activities

   1.   1.

   2.   2.

   3.   3.

   4.   4.

C. With the same student in mind, list what specific lan-
    guage comprehension/listening strategies need to be
    taught. What are some additional activities for teach-
    ing them?

           Specific Strategies   Activities

        1.   1.

        2.   2.

        3.   3.

        4.   4.

D. With the same student in mind, list appropriate commer-
    cial programs/resources. What elements of these programs/
    resources are best suited for teaching this student? What
    elements are least important?

        1.

        2.

        3.

        4.

INTERVENTION STRATEGIES:

LANGUAGE PRODUCTION/CONVERSATIONAL SKILLS

I. INTRODUCTION

Talking is one of the most effective and efficient methods by which we communicate. Students who have difficulty communicating verbally are at an extreme disadvantage in a society that values communication. This section is designed to first, present what to teach the adolescent who is having difficulty in the area of language production/conversational skills, and second, how to teach those skills.

II. WHAT TO TEACH

Adequate use of linguistic features, paralinguistic features, and conversational acts are goals for students with deficits. Specific behaviors within each of these areas have been cited in the "What to Assess" section of Language Production/Conversational Skills. Activities to enhance many of these skills are included in the next section, III B.

III. HOW TO TEACH

This section is divided into three areas: General Strategies; Specific Strategies for selected language production/conversational skills; and Commercially Available Programs and/or Resources that may be used to teach students with language disorders.

A. General Strategies for Language Production/Conversational Skills

1. Teaching Order

In the past, we concerned ourselves with whether students could, first of all, articulate sounds of the language, then combine sounds into words, then words into sentences. Later we began to examine whether those sentences were meaningful to others around the speaker, and recently, we have addressed the functional value and appropriateness of these utterances. As a general strategy, this order can be reversed during the intervention process with adolescents with language disorders. Establishing the functional value of the skills being taught is essential. Until the student recognizes the need for, or value in, acquiring a new language production/conversational skill, there will be little motivation to achieve a set objective. The following questions can be asked when setting intervention goals for language production/conversational skills with students:

182

a. In your opinion, what skills are most important for you to learn?

b. Why is it important that these skills be learned?

c. Where or in what situation would you need these skills?

d. How do you think we could proceed to help you learn the skill?

Involving the adolescent in intervention decisions and in taking ownership for his/her disorder in language production is necessary before any specific strategies can be applied. Students may resist exploring the answers to the questions above. They are more accustomed to listening and being told what to do rather than discussing their problems and focusing upon increasing their verbal skills.

2. <u>Conversational Skills</u>

At all times during the intervention process, the rules for conversation need to be followed. Regardless of the specific paths or activities being used, general strategies for conversation should be followed.

a. Have the students use clear conversational speech (Grice, 1975).

   i. The students should make informative contributions, but no more informative than necessary.

   ii. The students should not make what they believe to be false statements or make statements for which they lack adequate evidence.

   iii. The students' conversational comments should be relevant.

   iv. The students should avoid obscurity and ambiguity, and should be brief and orderly.

b. The students should be polite during their conversational speech (Grice, 1975).

   i. The students should not impose on their listeners.

   ii. The students should give options to their listeners.

      iii. The students should be friendly and make a listener feel comfortable.

  c. If there are two participants, both students have turns at speaking. If more than two people are participating, students do not need to take turns at speaking (Rees and Wollner, 1982).

  d. Only one speaker speaks at a time (usually). If two or more students start simultaneously, all but one drop out (Rees and Wollner, 1982).

  e. Participants who are not speaking pay attention to the one who is speaking. Attention is indicated by turning toward and/or looking at the speaker, not interrupting, acknowledging understanding of the speaker by gestural or verbal cues (e.g., "uh-huh"), or performing an action related to the content of the speaker's utterance (Rees and Wollner, 1982).

  f. Silent gaps between speakers' turns are brief or nonexistent and transitions are orderly (Rees and Wollner, 1982).

It is recommended that conversational rules be discussed during the intervention process, posted in the room, and referred to as necessary throughout all other remediation activities.

3. <u>Basic Skills Guidelines</u> for speaking skills are becoming available from more and more states. Referring again to Vermont's (1977) example of minimum skills expected from high school graduates, the following skills are emphasized:

  a. The students should give clear and accurate directions for reaching a selected location.

  b. The students should demonstrate organization, sequence, clarity, and accuracy when giving directions, explaining a process, making a report, or expressing an opinion.

  c. In a simulated situation, the students should demonstrate the ability to answer a business telephone correctly and take a message.

  d. The students should demonstrate the ability to get information or assistance by using the telephone.

  e. The students should demonstrate the ability to introduce themselves to others.

f. The students should respond to questions in an interview about their qualifications, experiences, and interests, and should ask relevant questions.

g. The students should participate, listen to others, make suitable responses, and speak loudly and clearly enough to be heard by all with whom they are communicating.

You may wish to check with your state to see what is currently being suggested with regard to curriculum goals in the area of speaking. A number of states are publishing guides for use by secondary school personnel. Some of their general strategies may be applicable to adolescents with language disorders.

B. Specific Strategies for Selected Language Production/Conversational Skills

1. Goals and Activities for Appropriate Production of Linguistic Features of the Language

a. Improve Production of Complex Sentences

Tasks suggested in the Listening section concerning complex sentences asked the students to judge whether complex sentences were complete or incomplete. It was also suggested that students break complex sentences into their underlying component sentences. Production of complex sentences can be facilitated as follows:

i. Have the student synthesize component sentences. For example:

-- The girl is happy.
-- The girl just found her lost cat.
-- The girl who just found her lost cat is happy.

-- The dog was licking the bowl.
-- The dog is my neighbor's.
-- The dog that was licking the bowl is my neighbor's.

ii. Have the student identify in what linguistic context it is appropriate to use "who" or "whom," and in which context it is appropriate to use "that," "what," or "which."

iii. Have the student explain the underlying meaning of a complex sentence. Question the student until you are certain he/she has attached meaning to that sentence.

185

b. Improve Production of Conjoined Sentences

Tasks suggested in the Listening section concerning conjoined sentences asked the students to judge whether conjoined sentences were complete or incomplete. It was also suggested that students break conjoined sentences into their underlying component sentences. Production of conjoined sentences can be facilitated as follows:

i.   Have the student complete an incomplete conjoined sentence with a specific phrase that would be appropriate. For example:

-- You have a choice of a baked potato, hash browns, _____.

ii. Have the student participate in cloze procedures in which they provide a critical word which was deleted from the sentence. For example:

-- I am taking my swimming suit with me _____ the hotel has a pool.

iii. Have the student paraphrase conjoined sentences. For example:

-- Because it is cloudy outside, I can't decide what to wear.

iv. Have the student form sentences using specific conjunctions. For example:

-- Produce a sentence that includes the word <u>although</u>.

v.   Have the student synthesize two sentences into a conjoined sentence. For example:

-- I am not going. I hate sitting through concerts.

c. Improve Production of Multiple-Meaning Words

i.   Have the student identify words that have multiple meanings within sentences. For example:

-- How can the word "can" be used within a sentence?

ii. Have the student generate a number of sentences upon being given a multiple-meaning
word. For example:

-- Upon being given the word <u>play</u>, have the
    student create several sentences in which
    that word would have a different meaning.

iii. Have the student identify what grammatical
roles a multiple-meaning word can play (e.g.,
"ship"). Also have the student identify how
this word changes grammatical form as prefixes and suffixes are added (e.g., "shipless").

d. Improve Production of Question Forms

i. Have the student participate in cloze procedures providing the critical question word
within a sentence. For example:

-- _____ will the show end?

Also have the student discuss whether the
blank can be completed with one WH-word or
whether several choices could be appropriate.

ii. Have the student participate in direct sentence transformation. For example:

-- You don't know him very well.

Ask a question with the same words.

iii. Have the student generate appropriate questions for specific situations. For example:

-- How would you find out if your friends
   could go with you to the movie tonight?

iv. Have the student generate several questions
that will result in the same answer. For
example:

-- When does the class get over?
-- What time does the class get over?

When first beginning this task, one question
could be provided for the student and the
other generated by the student. Later, the
situation only can be presented.

v. Have the student provide questions that match
specific answers (e.g., "Jeopardy Game" style).

e. Improve Production of Negation

    i. Have the student describe the relationship between the negation word (e.g., no, not) and the word or phrase that is negated within the sentence.

    ii. Have the student listen to sentences containing double negations, and restate the sentence using correct grammatical form. For example:

        -- They don't have no books.
        -- They don't have any books.

    iii. Have the student explain why some sentences can tolerate the appearance of two (or three) negation words within the sentence. For example:

        -- I don't know where the "No Smoking" sign is.
        -- His not going isn't going to change my mind.
        -- Just because I won't doesn't mean you can't.

    iv. Have the student express disagreement or refuse a request, in an appropriate manner.

f. Improve Production of Vocabulary

During the assessment of language production, it is important to have determined whether the student's lack of vocabulary is due to a restricted choice of words or to word retrieval problems (i.e., the student has the vocabulary, but cannot recall it on demand). Intervention strategies are vastly different, depending upon whether the emphasis is increasing vocabulary or giving the student cueing strategies for retrieving words that are already acquired. This section shall address the student who has a restricted choice of words. Section "g," which immediately follows, will describe word retrieval strategies. Appropriate activities to improve vocabulary production follow:

    i. Have the student group new vocabulary words by categories. Hall (1976) has called this the establishment of "semantic maps." Connecting new words to those already within one's vocabulary makes the task of retaining new vocabulary much easier. For some students, this may involve going back to some cognitive tasks that emphasize classification and categorization, as well as hierarchical classification (e.g., neighborhood, community, town, city, county, state, nation, continent).

   ii. Have the student define meanings for common prefixes and suffixes (e.g., prefixes: re-, un-, dis-, di-; suffixes: -ly, -less, -ful).

  iii. Have the student determine what prefixes or suffixes can be combined with certain root words (e.g., When combined with the root word "sight," in- is appropriate, but un- is not.)

   iv. Have the student participate in cloze procedures using sentences in which several appropriate derived forms of the same root word must be used. For example:

       -- After the windstorm, the town looked generally disorganized.
       -- After the last election, the voting districts were reorganized.

    v. Have the student create a visual connection with a new vocabulary word whenever possible. For example, heredity has as its dominant syllable "red." The student could establish a visual imagery of a huge red field swarming with genes and chromosomes which would help trigger the meaning of the word heredity. Usually, the more bizarre the image, the easier it is for the student to conjure up that image and, thus, the word or meaning of the word.

g. Increase Word Retrieval Skills

   The following strategies are taken from the work of Wiig and Semel (1980):

    i. Have the student name the conceptual category to which the intended word(s) belong(s) (e.g., "car" for Chevrolet).

   ii. Have the student identify the first letter and/or sound of the word to be retrieved. Make certain he/she is completing a systematic search of the alphabet.

iii. Have the student describe the physical characteristics and/or functions of an object. Description through use of negation may be helpful. For example:

-- It's not as big as a motorcycle, but it has a motor.

iv. Have the student use homonyms or synonyms for cues. Homonyms should be tried before synonyms. Antonyms can also be used.

v. Have the student use gestures, pretended actions, or other nonverbal cues to retrieve the word.

vi. Have the student use visual imagery to facilitate retrieval as described in the section above on vocabulary.

vii. Provide multiple word choices and have the student select the appropriate word. For example:

-- Is it a dog, a bike, or a tail?

viii. Have the student name a series of objects within a category, gradually attempting to increase speed.

ix. Have the student complete simple statements with a wide variety of possible words. For example:

-- I can eat _____.
-- My friends are _____.

This same task can be specifically directed to particular categories of words. For example, if the category is geographical locations, the following sentence could be used:

-- On vacation we always enjoy driving to _____.

x. Have the student participate in word association tasks. For example:

-- Name as many vehicles as you can in the next minute.

Again, these tasks can be specifically directed to desired relationships. For example, if focusing on temporal sequential relationships, the student could be asked to tell what comes before and after "June," "Winter," and "Monday."

Word retrieval cues may initially be supplied by adults interacting with the student, but the ultimate goal is to have the student develop self-cueing strategies that permit independent functioning.

2. <u>Goals and Activities for Appropriate Use of the Functions of Language</u>

   Simon (1980) suggested intervention strategies based upon the functions proposed by Halliday (1975).

   a. Improve Use of the Instrumental Function

      i. Have the student tell what he/she wants by use of a particular label.

      ii. Have the student identify polite versus impolite requests.

      iii. Have the student describe an object, using precise adjectives and prepositional modifiers. Have the student provide as much information as the situation demands.

      iv. Have the student analyze the communicative context and provide the amount of information necessary.

      v. Have the student request information in a polite manner in a role playing situation.

   b. Improve Use of the Regulatory Function

      i. Have the student demonstrate ability to use language to control behavior. For example:

         -- Please, do as I tell you.

      ii. Rather than using physical force to get his/her way, have the student use regulatory language.

      iii. Instead of engaging in tattling when involved in a peer confrontation, have the student use regulatory language.

iv. Have the student use the regulatory language function in role playing situations
(e.g., convincing a small child not to
play near the street, confronting someone
who tries to cut in front of you in a
line, telling someone a game has already
begun so he/she cannot play).

v. Have the student provide precise, sequenced
instruction for the reproduction of an
arrangement of objects.

c. Improve Use of the Interactional Function

i. Have the student demonstrate an ability to
analyze social situations, decide upon the
most effective communication behaviors,
and display them during role playing.

ii. In an informal discussion, have the student demonstrate that he/she can cope with
an adverse social situation using words
rather than physical force.

d. Improve Use of the Personal Function

i. Have the student formulate descriptive sentences about his/her individuality.

ii. Have the student express his/her likes or
dislikes when looking at pictures of food,
activity, careers, etc.

iii. Have the student express a value judgment
on three issues listed by the clinician
and critique them in terms of how they
meet specified moral criteria.

iv. Have the student present an opinion about
three community and three school rules.
Discuss alternative rules in terms of how
well they would meet specified moral criteria.

v. Have the student choose a quantified value
(all, some, no) and provide sufficient evidence to support that choice.

vi. Have the student present a 3-4 minute persuasive speech that displays at least three
pieces of evidence that supports his/her
position.

     vii. Have the student present an organized argu-
ment to support one side of a controversial
issue in a debate.

e. Improve the Use of the Heuristic Function

       i. Have the student generate at least 1-4
WH-questions about a picture, with or without prompts from an adult.

     ii. Have the student create enough significant
probes (WH- and yes-no questions) to formulate a hypothesis about the identity of a
mystery item.

   iii. Have the student listen to directives for
the placement of objects, ask questions to
clarify the directives, and determine when
he/she has sufficient information.

    iv. Have the student analyze vague directives
and formulate necessary clarification questions.

     v. Have the student spontaneously ask at least
10 questions to learn more about:

      -- The content of photographs

      -- Unfamiliar people and events

      -- A scientific experiment

      -- A Piagetian task

      -- The function of a mechanical object

    vi. Have the student formulate a certain number
of questions during a 30-minute session,
probing values and disvalues stated by his/
her peers.

   vii. Have the student ask questions that challenge the premises and conclusions of syl-
logisms or the efficacy of basic living
rules.

f. Improve Use of the Imaginative Function

       i. Have the student look at a picture and
create a story line that includes a beginning, middle, and end, with or without support from an adult.

ii. Have the student describe, provide dialogue for, or act out a given imaginary scene.

iii. In a team project with peers, have the student create a short story from an introductory phrase or sentence.

g. Improve Use of the Informational Function

i. During a therapy session, have the student describe a picture, him/herself, a problem, sensory impressions, etc.

ii. Have the student compare or contrast colors, categories, words, opinions, customs, careers, etc.

iii. Have the student explain the definition of multiple-meaning words, sports terms, figurative language, an activity, or an experiment.

iv. Have the student hypothesize about a problem, task, experiment, etc.

v. Have the student analyze a problem, story, part-whole relationship, etc.

vi. Have the student demonstrate inductive and deductive reasoning.

vii. Have the student evaluate a story, problem, opinion, value, and moral behavior.

C. Commercially Available Programs/Resources

1. Curriculum Guide Speech-Language Program - Secondary Level (D.C. Everest Public Schools, 1980)

The speech-language pathologists in D.C. Everest Public Schools developed a curriculum guide that includes major sections on language production, basic life skills, and pragmatics. Each section of the guide is then broken down into the following organizational scheme:

a. Specific Objectives

For example, an objective within the language production section is, "The student will select, retrieve, and use words effectively and efficiently in accordance with accepted word meanings while interacting with persons in the environment."

b. Content (Concepts/Skills Taught)

Under content for the objective cited above, these concepts are listed:

    i. Expansion of core/basic vocabulary

    ii. Use of antonyms, synonyms, and homonyms

    iii. Use of multiple meanings of words

    iv. Discretionary use of words having "shades of meaning," differentiation

c. Instructional Activities (Examples)

In addition to the specific objectives and content, example activities are listed in the curriculum guide. The following example is used for an instructional activity related to the information given above. "Student uses a word in at least two sentences demonstrating knowledge of its multiple meanings." For example:

-- He set the table for supper.

-- They voted to table the discussion.

-- She checked the water table.

The curriculum guide is available at a nominal charge by writing to D.C. Everest Public Schools, Schofield, Wisconsin 54476 (Attention: Director of Special Education).

2. Communicative Competence: A Functional-Pragmatic Approach to Language Therapy (Simon, 1980)

Simon's complete program includes her monograph, a teaching manual, four filmstrips, photo-diagram book, spinners, and stimulus cards. The manual suggests strategies that are useful with adolescents who have restricted syntax or are whom Simon labels "marginal communicators." Simon cites these major objectives for her program:

a. To have the client develop non-egocentric communication skills

b. To have the client establish rudimentary and refined syntactic and pragmatic skills so that messages are structurally correct, coherent, and composed of sufficient information for the listener

c. To have the professional develop an operational model of competent versus incompetent communication skills in the client

Excellent strategies are suggested, each rooted in functional use during daily living situations.

3. Source Book of Language Learning Activities: Instructional Strategies and Methods (Worthley, 1978)

The source book presents teaching techniques, a criterion placement test, and actual language activities for a wide range of communicative abilities. Some of the tests described would be appropriate at junior high levels (e.g., associating ideas, making comparisons, coordinating transformations, making two sentences into one, or making one sentence into two). However, the majority of the activities presented are too low-level unless used with very severely disordered secondary students.

4. HELP: Handbook of Exercises for Language Processing, Volumes I and II (Lazzari and Peters, 1981)

The two HELP books are designed to improve auditory processing skills and language processing skills through the use of exercises relevant to daily living. The authors suggest their tasks are suitable for ages 6 through adult and can be used by teachers, paraprofessionals, and parents. The handbooks are filled with actual sentences and lists that can be used during intervention sessions and are, thus, a great time saver.

Topics addressed include WH-questions, specific word-finding, auditory reception, and auditory association, to name a few.

5. Lifestyles (Lozano and Sturtevant, 1981)

Although Lifestyles is actually an intermediate level course in English, it is function-based and its intent is to have students learn to understand spoken, natural discourse. It also helps students learn to communicate in work, social, and academic situations. Reading and writing activities are included within Lifestyles, but it would also be feasible to use the oral communication activities from the curriculum as part of the intervention process.

6. Sense and Nonsense, a Study in Human Communication (Fleishman, 1971) and Troubled Talk! (Fleishman, 1973)

Alfred Fleishman, the author of these two books, is actually from the Public Relations field, but has spent a considerable amount of time and energy applying the principles of communication to everyday living. A number of the ideas presented in his publications would be useful as springboards for discussion with language disordered adolescents. He has called his second book "a practical guide to improving language habits." Some of the bad language habits he suggests we change include interrupting each other, imposing our views on each other, and saying that we know all about something. He goes on to suggest strategies for overcoming these difficulties in communication.

7. Communications: The Transfer of Meaning (Sabun, 1968)

This book provides a brief summation of communication principles as they apply to everyday life. It could be helpful resource in beginning intervention with conversational skills at the junior/senior high school level. Sabun discusses communication in terms of input, processing, and output. His discussion closely resembles the cognitive model of input-elaboration-output addressed in the works of Reuven Feuerstein. A number of intervention goals and activities could be built around basic ideas presented in this book.

8. Making Sense: Exploring Semantics and Critical Thinking (Potter, 1974)

Although written more as a textbook for adolescent students, this book is one of the few that emphasizes oral communication skills. Numerous activities addressing language production and conversational skills can be adapted within a speech-language intervention program. Attention is focused more on accurate and appropriate transmission of messages than on grammatical form.

9. Human Communication Handbook: Simulations and Games Volume I (Ruben & Budd, 1975) and Volume II (Ruben, 1978)

These handbooks describe many useful adolescent group activities for improving conversational skills and language function. The activities are designed to engage the participants in specific speaking situations followed by discussions for insight. For example, one activity called "Rumor: Serial Transmission of Information" requires a number of participants to leave the room while the others watch an action film. One by one, the group members who had left are brought back into the room as information about the film is shared. This activity focuses upon the process of transmitting verbal information in serial fashion and the errors that are likely to occur. Many activities emphasize interpersonal communication and group dynamics. Each of the handbooks addresses topics of intrapersonal, social, cross-cultural/intercultural, and mass communication.

10. A Handbook of Verbal Group Exercises (Morris and Cinnamon, 1974)

   Many activities focusing upon language production/conversational skills are presented in this handbook. Most of them are designed to be used with groups rather than individuals. Tasks are described under such category headings as Communication, Consensus, Empathy, and Rejection. Since many of the activities focus on personal awareness and growth and social-emotional growth, the adult planning the intervention strategies would need to carefully select and/or adapt activities to meet the objectives established for students.

11. Let's Talk: Developing Prosocial Communication Skills (Wiig, 1982)

   This material can be used to meet social communication needs in adolescents with language disorders. The complete program includes:

   a. A manual which features background materials and communication skill training activities

   b. Five communication card games emphasizing communication skills in functional situations and context

   c. Functional Communicational Score Sheets

   d. Four communication card games emphasizing different communication intents

   e. Communication Intents Score Sheets

   The card games were designed to be used with standard cards or in role-playing formats with small groups. Wiig has suggested that the material can be used with persons from 9 to 21 years of age.

12. Thematic Language Simulation (Morganstein and Smith, 1982)

   This is a workbook designed for aphasics, and is built upon topic units such as sports, transportation, cooking, and weather. Many of the suggested activities

198

could also be adapted for use with language disordered adolescents. The workbook includes more than 300 reproducible worksheets. Some of the tasks that seem particularly adaptable to adolescents include categorization of words, sentence arrangement, and sentence correction.

13. Workbook for Aphasia (Brubaker, 1978)

Described as "exercises for the redevelopment of higher level language functioning," this workbook presents activities that could be adapted for use with adolescents. For example, the section on "Use of Factual Information" focuses upon WH-questions and provides extensive lists of questions that could be used with adolescents. The workbook format calls for many written responses, but it could easily be modified to an oral format.

14. Sentence Solitaire (Mullica, 1982)

Common sentence constructions can be built with seven card decks, 200 cards in all. Activities suggested in this material are based on the familiar game of Solitaire. Since it was developed with adults in mind, the pictures on the cards are appropriate to use with older students. Constructions that can be built include the following:

a. Noun + Verb

b. Noun + Verb + Noun

c. Noun + Verb + Preposition + Noun

15. Concepts for Communication Series (Wright, Norris, and Worsley, 1974)

This curriculum series is based upon referential communication activities to be used with students working in pairs. Some of the actual materials in Concepts for Communication will be too childish for older adolescents, but the activity format is an excellent orientation for educators who have not previously used referential communication games. These games include fixed arrays of pictures, sets of pictures placed in a particular location, maps that can be used when describing directions, models that can be described and built, and symbols that can be drawn.

16. <u>Development and Intervention with the Hearing Impaired</u>
(Kretschner, Jr. and Kretschner, 1978)

Although focused on the hearing-impaired population, this book contains a wealth of information applicable to older students without hearing problems. The authors provide an extensive outline of sequences for teaching developmental language. These sequences are presented in a table format that includes advanced structures such as subordinate conjunctions, relative clauses, and passives. They have also suggested a number of general educational procedures to consider with language disordered students.

IV. <u>SUMMARY</u>

This section presents information on the importance of teaching language production/conversational skills, what to teach, and how to teach it. In the discussion of how to teach the student, the authors present general strategies, specific strategies for selected tasks, and available commercial programs and resources.

V. ACTIVITIES

A. Select one student currently on your caseload and list in order of priority the language production/conversational goals for this student.

1.

2.

3.

4.

B. With the same student in mind, list which general language production/conversational strategies he/she needs to learn. What are some additional activities for teaching them?

General Strategies   Activities

1.   1.

2.   2.

3.   3.

4.   4.

C. With the same student in mind, list what specific language production/conversational strategies need to be
   taught. What are some additional activities for teaching them?

                Specific Strategies   Activities

        1.   1.

        2.   2.

        3.   3.

        4.   4.

D. With the same student in mind, list appropriate commercial programs/resources. What elements of these programs/
   resources are best suited for teaching this student?
   What elements are least important?

        1.

        2.

        3.

        4.

INTERVENTION STRATEGIES: SURVIVAL LANGUAGE SKILLS

I. INTRODUCTION

It is critical that students develop adequate speech and
language skills for use in daily living situations if they
are to be integrated into the surrounding community. Appropriate communication with family, friends, and co-workers is
essential to survival in the world beyond the school walls.

II. WHAT TO TEACH

A. Prerequisite Skills

1. If it is determined that prerequisite work in the
    area of concepts and operations needs to be pur-
    sued, the reader may wish to refer to the "Interven-
    tion Strategies: Cognitive Skills" section.

2. Adequate survival language skills mean that the stu-
    dent has a minimal ability to successfully partici-
    pate in informative and critical listening activities.
    The reader is urged to refer to the intervention sec-
    tion addressing language comprehension/listening if
    prerequisite skills are needed in this area.

3. At the onset, the educator should recognize that the
    adolescent will need to memorize a minimum number of
    words as sight words in order to survive in our soci-
    ety. It is recommended that sight words be selected
    according to their relevance in the student's world
    and their urgency with regard to personal health and
    safety. For example, "danger" may be more critical
    for many than "open." While sight recognition is
    important, the actual comprehension of the word,
    whether spoken or printed, is absolutely critical.
    "Reading" the word without attaching meaning continues
    to leave the adolescent without survival language
    skills.

4. In addition to words, there has been an increasingly
    larger number of symbols (rebuses) developed to repre-
    sent objects, services, and rules. The trend has
    moved toward universality of symbols. It is as impor-
    tant to derive meaning from these symbols as from the
    sight word vocabulary emphasized above. If, for example,
    the student is not aware that signs with a slash mark
    through them indicate "no," then comprehension of that
    rebus would be a prerequisite to understanding many
    signs utilizing that mark.

B. Compensatory Strategies

Time is of the essence with secondary level students with speech-language disorders. Some students and circumstances may indicate that spending time on prerequisite skills is unwise, unnecessary, or not in the best interests of the student. For example, blind people, who certainly cannot read signs and labels surrounding them, can probably ask questions about them and persuade people who do read to help them. Thus, a compensatory strategy might involve teaching students with language disorders to ask specific questions about what they cannot read and/or understand.

Consider the student who has definite deficits in quantity concepts and numerical operations. If time is of the essence, would it not be better to train him/her to use a calculator rather than the underlying strategies of long division?

Whether to insist on underlying prerequisites or to forge ahead and substitute compensatory strategies is a decision that needs to be made with the student. One senior in high school recently balked at the idea of knowing about food packaging labels and cooking directions. After all, he was going to find a wife who did all that so why should he bother to learn? (Such a "compensatory strategy" was determined to not be in his best interests in the long run!)

III. HOW TO TEACH

This section is divided into two areas: General Strategies for Teaching Survival Language Skills and Commercially Available Programs and/or Resources.

A. General Strategies for Teaching Survival Language Skills

It is recommended that the following methodology be used to personally design survival language skills intervention:

1. Develop a general objective(s). A general objective is the long-range focus of a functional, practical curriculum. Valletutti and Bender (1982) give this example of a long-term objective: "The individual will function as a traveler in the local and greater community as skillfully and as independently as possible."

2. Jointly plan specific objectives stated in behavioral terms. Whenever possible, the criterion should be set for natural settings and real-life context. For example, "The student will independently plan, schedule, and take a trip on the city bus when he needs to travel some place out of walking distance."

204

3. Determine cognitive dimensions inherent in the task. For example, have the student estimate the time needed to catch the bus or identify streets on a map. Also, determine if the student(s) has any physical attributes that would make it difficult for him/her to achieve the objective (e.g., the student is on crutches and would need to allow extra time to catch the bus). It may also be helpful to discuss any health and safety factors with the students to make them aware of any dangers (e.g., avoiding sites with warnings such as "Do Not Enter," "No Trespassing").

4. Introduce the vocabulary words for the overall unit. Determine this vocabulary by completing a task analysis of what needs to occur for the student to go from the current level of performance to achieving the specific objective. For example, if the focus is going to be on travel by car, bus, and airplane, the student(s) would be provided with vocabulary that addresses that topic.

5. Categorize the vocabulary by one or more strategies (e.g., "what is common to all travel and what is unique to each mode of travel").

6. Introduce initial materials needed to complete the objective, in this case the bus schedule and route map. It may be a store layout, sample labels, various clocks, or a teletrainer.

7. Role-play the situation (e.g., planning, scheduling, and taking a trip on the bus).

8. Present problem solving situations (e.g., "what if this happened....").

9. Take a field trip or in another way immerse the student in the desired situation. Discuss the field trip. What was learned? What is left to be learned?

10. Have the student independently complete a similar field trip. Determine whether the specific objective was met. If not, repeat role playing, problem solving, and field trip experiences. Analyze the student's performance to determine what behaviors are preventing the achievement of the terminal objective.

B. Comercially Available Programs/Resources

1. Survival Vocabularies (Richey, 1978) and Sign Language: A Survival Vocabulary (Richey, 1977) provide excellent resource data on topics such as the language of the supermarket, of restaurants, and of entertainment, and warning signs such as "handle with care" and "swim at your own risk." Although unique in their pulling together of survival words, the books are not unique in their strategies for teaching the vocabulary. However, the knowledgeable educator could easily use the vocabulary and design appropriate tasks for the adolescent to learn the words in context.

2. Survival Guides (1977) are published by Jannus Book Publishers and range in topic from "Getting Around Cities and Towns" to "Reading Schedules" to "Using the Want Ads." Again, their primary value for intervention probably rests most heavily on the specialized survival vocabulary identified for each topic. The same publisher also prints a number of publications regarding jobs -- applying for them, interviewing for them, and holding them.

3. Teaching Interpersonal and Community Living Skills: A Curriculum Model for Handicapped Adolescents and Adults (Valletutti and Bender, 1982) and Teaching Functional Academics: A Curriculum Guide for Adolescents and Adults with Learning Problems (Bender and Valletutti, 1982) are excellent resources for planning objectives in the area of survival language skills. They emphasize the need for educators to diligently examine the functional reality of a stated objective. If there is no functional essence, any objectives or instructional acts become impractical.

   At the end of both texts, there are excellent sections of "Selected References" that provide a wealth of information to the reader.

4. Teletrainer equipment is available at no charge from the Bell Telephone Company. Through prior arrangement, they will allow the use of a telephone training kit for a specified time period. The kit is independent of the phone system, yet allows actual phone conversations to be conducted. Teletrainer equipment is vital to teaching a unit on survival telephone language.

5. Curriculum Analysis and Design for Retarded Learners
   (Klein, Pasch, and Frew, 1979)

   The final chapter in this book, "Analyzing Curriculum
   Materials," presents an excellent list of resources
   for a functional life curriculum. Countless commercial products are available that focus on topics such
   as housekeeping, family living, money management, and
   production and consumption of foods and services to
   name just a few. The reader will be amazed at the
   vast amount of information that can be adapted for use
   during survival language skill intervention.

III. SUMMARY

   This section presents information on the importance of teaching survival language skills, what to teach, and how to teach
   it. In the discussion of how to teach the student, the authors
   present general strategies, specific strategies for selected
   tasks, and available commercial programs and resources.

IV. ACTIVITIES

    A. Select one student currently on your caseload and list
       in order of priority the major survival language goals
       for this student.

       1.

       2.

       3.

       4.

    B. With the same student in mind, list which general sur-
       vival language strategies he/she needs to learn. What
       are some additional activities for teaching them?

          General Strategies   Activities

       1.   1.

       2.   2.

       3.   3.

       4.   4.

C. With the same student in mind, list what specific survival
   language strategies need to be taught. What are some additional activities for teaching them?

        Specific Strategies   Activities

1.   1.

2.   2.

3.   3.

4.   4.

D. With the same student in mind, list appropriate commercial programs/resources. What elements of these pro-
   grams/resources are best suited for teaching this student? What elements are least important?

1.

2.

3.

4.

INTERVENTION STRATEGIES: EDUCATIONAL SYSTEM

I. ## INTRODUCTION

When intervention with the curriculum is considered, it can be accomplished in one of two ways:

A. The curriculum can be modified to fit the existing performance of the student.

B. The existing performance of the student can be modified to fit the curriculum.

The authors believe it is critical that junior/senior high school students learn to adapt to the environment around them. At some point in the near future, it will no longer be possible for someone to take them by the hand and modify the world to fit their particular needs and wants. Therefore, when intervention with the curriculum occurs, it is primarily to equip the student with the necessary language skills and strategies to survive. This is accomplished through intervention strategies suggested in the previous sections of this manual. However, there may be particular situations and students for whom intervention with the language of instruction (textbook and instructor) is desirable. This section addresses modifications that might be made within the curriculum for the adolescent with language disorders.

II. ## WHAT TO TEACH

Modifications in the curriculum to better meet a student's needs may include:

A. Adapting printed information to the language level of the student

B. Providing alternative input or output modalities that emphasize the student's strengths

C. Training educators to more effectively communicate with adolescents who have language disorders.

III. ## HOW TO TEACH

This section is divided into General Strategies for Modifying Curriculum, Specific Strategies that can be utilized for deficiencies identified with the CALI, and Commercial Programs/ Resources.

A. General Strategies for Modifying Curriculum

1. Awareness and Ownership

Often the adult(s) in the language disordered student's world will modify the curriculum without that person's knowledge. Modifications are not discussed with the student, and may not even be within his/her awareness level. The authors recommend a general strategy that includes student awareness of the curriculum modifications made, and encourages gradual student ownership of the responsibility for those modifications. If, for example, the modification was one of highlighting the main ideas in a chapter, it would be advantageous for the student to learn the process of identifying and highlighting these ideas. The ultimate goal would be for students to develop their own strategies for modifying and simplifying the information they are to process.

2. Teacher Self-Evaluation

The following checklist can be provided to teachers of language disordered adolescents who are willing to evaluate their personal language of instruction:

a. Do I speak in complete, uninterrupted sentences?

b. How many points do I make in each sentence?

c. Do I guard against using words or concepts beyond the student's understanding?

d. Is my speaking voice, rate, and volume satisfactory?

e. When asking a question, do I ask the question and then call upon the student, or do I call upon the student and then ask the question?

f. Is my attention centered on student reaction while giving instructions or directions?

g. Do I watch for indications revealing that the student no longer understands what is being said?

h. When misunderstanding occurs, do I restate my question or directions in a different way or repeat what I formerly said?

i. When I use visual aids or a pointer, are my movements precise and definite?

j. Am I aware of any distracting influences in the classroom?

k. Do I have everyone's individual attention before asking a question or making an explanation?

l. Am I aware of personal habits which might prove distracting to the class?

m. Do I use specific instances and illustrations as an aid to understanding?

n. Does my question require a factual answer or an answer based on critical thinking?

o. Do I facilitate student understanding by asking questions in a sequence leading them to a conclusion I want them to reach?

p. Do I allow time for students to assimilate what has been said before moving on to the next point?

3. Adapting and Enhancing Language in the Classroom (Wiig and Semel, 1980)

This book states that all language used in classroom instruction may have to be adapted or enhanced to allow the language disordered student to function optionally in the regular classroom. Modifications they suggest include the following:

a. If the content or structure of material is new or unfamiliar to the student, sentences should be spoken at a rate slower than normal conversational speech.

b. Intonation patterns, phrasing, and stress should not be different from that within normal conversational speech.

c. Order-of-mention information, directions, or computations need to be sequenced in the order of action required for execution.

d. Information that is to be recalled later should be compiled in a list and given to the student. This list can be used for reference and questioning. Lists of definitions and illustrations are also recommended. (Note: The authors would advise that adolescent students assume some responsibility for the development of these lists as the intervention process proceeds.)

e. Contents of materials and presentations should be provided in outline form for the students.

f. Taperecordings, particularly of written instructions or materials, may be helpful to the students. Taperecording may also replace note-taking.

g. A buddy system may be established in which students with different, but complementary, abilities assist each other with classroom assignments.

h. Sentence length of from 5-8 words may be helpful.

i. WH-questions may be rephrased into simpler language (e.g., "who" is rephrased into "what person").

j. Untimed tests are often more valid than timed tests. Taperecordings of spoken responses to test items may be considered for some students.

B. Specific Strategies

1. Familiarity with Textbook

   Have the student become familiar with any features of the textbook that were identified with the CALI (e.g., given the topic word "prepositional phrase," what feature of the textbook would most quickly tell you the pages that address that topic). If the textbook contains features which the student does not know how to use, have the student generate a definition, a rationale for its inclusion, and an example of when the feature would be used.

2. Comprehension of the Specific Vocabulary of the Curriculum

   Intervention strategies are contained within the listening section that addresses comprehension of lectures. While it is essential to isolate the specific vocabulary and concept deficits surfacing in the curriculum, it is equally important to not become a tutor to the student in a particular content area. The focus is one of providing a strategy for learning new vocabulary, not on the new words per se. The focus is on generalizing those strategies, not on narrowing the terminology to an isolated word list. See "Vocabulary" in Intervention Strategies: Language Production/Conversational Skills for general strategies. Comprehension of vocabulary will not always precede production of vocabulary. Sometimes the process is reversed or only partial comprehension is evident. This

213

is not unusual for any adolescent or adult language user. We often produce words without full knowledge of the meaning (e.g., "stock market," while generally known by many, is specifically comprehended by few). Having the student comprehend vocabulary specific to various curricula can be facilitated by:

a. Keeping a notebook and/or notecard file system for each subject. Students are responsible for stating definitions in their own words and reviewing frequently.

b. Highlighting new vocabulary in printed material. (Advocacy may be needed to convince administrators of the need to mark certain texts and printed material.)

c. Asking the teachers to provide lists of new vocabulary, or asking them to verify that the student's list is accurate. (Note that the responsible individual is the student, not the adult providing intervention services. Modeling and assistance may be provided initially.)

d. Connecting new vocabulary items with "old" familiar words. Connections may be provided through categorization, synonyms, antonyms, homonyms, analogies, visual imagery, etc. The emphasis is on linking what is unfamiliar with what is already known and remembered by the student.

C. Commercially Available Programs/Resources

1. Project Stile (1979)

With the assistance of Dr. Gordon Alley and Dr. Donald Deshler, a learning strategy for working with language-learning disabled adolescents was developed. The philosophical premises upon which Project Stile is based mesh closely with philosophical premises cited by the authors. When working with language-learning disabled adolescents, Alley and Deshler caution against the tutorial approach, the vocational approach, the compensatory approach, and the basic skills approach. Shortcomings of these approaches include an emphasis on course work rather than on underlying inability to learn; denial of the benefits of regular classroom curricula; failure to teach the adolescent how to cope with demands independently; and focusing on the traditional basic skills of "reading, writing, rithmetic," but not on the broader range of basic skills that need to include listening, speaking, and thinking.

214

In Project Stile, the overall objective is to have students "learn how to learn." The project does not recommend:

-- Changing the classroom expectations (unless they totally preclude success)

-- Watering down content

-- Teaching specific academic content

-- Teaching basic reading and mathematic skills beyond the functional (fourth-fifth grade) levels

The Project does recommend:

-- Determining what skills are needed for success in school and in life

-- Teaching as many of these as possible to a functional level

It also teaches how these skills can be used in a variety of situations and settings.

Instructional objectives and activities are provided for these crucial learning skills:

a. Study skills, including time management, textbook use, test skills, and visual aids

b. Reading skills, including skimming, scanning, and structural analysis

c. Listening skills, including listening comprehension at a literal level and a critical level

d. Writing skills, including note-taking and written expression

e. Thinking skills, including questioning, flow charting, and strategies for remembering

Adults planning intervention strategies for adolescents with language disorders would find a wealth of information from Project Stile.

2. Oklahoma Project (1982)

With regard to adapting the educational system, the Oklahoma Project provides an extensive description of modifications that can be made. Teachers are trained through a series of workshops to modify their textbooks

215

and classroom presentations so that students with language disorders and learning problems may grasp main ideas more easily. For example, all textbooks are color coded using the same system throughout the school. The model strongly promotes the SQ3R approach to reading and studying:

a. Survey -- Skim each page

b. Question -- Ask questions during skimming (e.g., "What is this about?")

c. Read -- Engage in the active process of decoding the material

d. Recite -- Close the book and think, "What did I read?"

e. Review -- Open the book and review again

Numerous dissemination products are available from the Oklahoma Project. Staff members from their center provide in-service training for schools which use their training model.

3. Program Development Assistance Systems (PDAS)

Located at the University of Washington - Seattle, PDAS provides current information on all model secondary programs in the country. Any project currently receiving federal monies to implement exemplary programs for adolescents is affiliated with that office. PDAS acts as a national clearinghouse for information and could provide current data on any projects addressing curriculum adaptation that involve grants from the federal level.

IV. SUMMARY

Many options exist for adapting the curriculum to students with language disorders and learning problems. Perhaps the basic question is, "How much do you want to adapt the environment to the student versus the student to the environment?" Several excellent curriculum projects (Project STILE and the Oklahoma Project) provide extensive information on adapting the educational system. Many of their ideas could be applied and at the same time, could work toward teaching the strategies to the students themselves.

V. ACTIVITIES

   A. Select a student who is on your caseload and in the main-
       stream, but who has difficulty with one or more subject
       areas. List ways that the curriculum could be modified
       to better meet his/her needs:

       1.

       2.

       3.

       4.

   B. Make a plan for initiating the changes indicated in "A"
       (i.e., How would you do it? Who would need to be involved?).

       1.

       2.

       3.

       4.

       5.

       6.

       7.

   C. With this same student in mind, list which skills he/she
       would need to acquire in order to adapt to the curriculum,
       rather than vice versa.

       1.

       2.

       3.

       4.

       5.

       6.

INTERVENTION STRATEGIES: ENVIRONMENTAL CONDITIONS

I. INTRODUCTION

Intervention strategies should include suggestions for both the family and peers of language disordered adolescents.

II. STRATEGIES FOR THE FAMILY

If there are problems within the family other than communication differences or disorders, we would recommend referral to the appropriate professional. Weekly, biweekly, or monthly conferences with family members are perhaps the most instructional, since they directly address their child's progress. Whenever possible, have the teen-ager accompany the parents to the conferences. However, we also recommend annual or biannual in-services on appropriate topics such as "What are Communication Disorders?", "Strategies to Enhance Listening Skills," "How to Talk and Listen to Your Teen-ager." If feasible, have a parent seminar where a number of parents of language disordered adolescents can come together to share common concerns, frustrations, and alternative solutions to problems. We strongly urge the formation of parent support groups. Such a group could provide a vehicle for counseling families and would assist parents in sorting out their concerns with and suggestions for working with their children with communication disorders. If there are older or younger siblings, they should be counseled regarding the impact of having a brother or sister with a language disorder. Also, they should be informed of ways they might assist the language disordered person.

III. STRATEGIES FOR THE PEERS

Peer relationships are extremely important to students at this age level. It is important to help peers of the student with a language disorder to understand what it means to have a communication handicap. We can do this by showing movies and involving them in activities which show what it is like to not be able to understand language and follow directions or lectures. It is important to not only talk to them about communication disorders, but also to help them experience, via simulated activities and discussions, what it might be like to have a language disorder.

IV. SUMMARY

It is essential to involve family members and peers of the language disordered adolescent in the intervention process if maximum progress is to be made. Ideally, this would take the form of group sessions that focus on information dissemination and/or counseling.

218

V. ACTIVITIES

    A. List meeting topics of interest to parents and peers of your adolescent students.

        1.

        2.

        3.

    B. List strategies for increasing parental interest and participation in activities such as in-services, conferences/interviews, and support groups.

        1.

        2.

        3.

GLOSSARY

GLOSSARY

ACTIVE VOICE - The subject/agent of a sentence is performing the action (e.g., The girl is saving the puppy.).

AUGMENTATIVE COMMUNICATION - A system used to supplement the communicative skills of individuals for whom speech is temporarily or permanently inadequate to meet communicative needs (ASHA, 1982).

AUXILIARY VERB - A verb form of have, be, or do; also includes the class of verbs called modals.

BASAL LEVEL - On a test, it is the level at which all items are passed. It immediately precedes the level where the first failure occurs. It is assumed that all items below the basal point are correct.

CEILING LEVEL - On a test, it is the highest item of a sequence in which a certain number of items has been failed. It is assumed all items above ceiling level are incorrect.

CENTRAL TENDENCIES - A statistical measure used to describe typical values in a set, or distribution of scores (Compton, 1980). The Mean, Median, and Mode are the most common measures used in educational testing.

CLOZE PROCEDURE - A format used in teaching and testing in which certain words are deleted from the text during reading or from the spoken language when talking, leaving a blank space for the student to fill. Determination is made of the number of blanks the students can accurately fill.

COGNITION - One's knowledge of the world. A mental process of knowing and becoming aware of the world.

CONCRETE OPERATIONAL PERIOD - The period of development in which the child has developed the operations of classification, seriation, and conservation. Thinking is now decentered and reversible. Inductive reasoning is present. Most children enter this period around seven years of age.

FORMAL OPERATIONAL PERIOD - The period in which a person engages in abstract thought and can use hypothetical-deductive reasoning. The person can now systematically control variables, can consider all possible combinations, can use proportionality and logic, and has an integrated system of operations. Most students make the transition to the formal period between 11 and 13 years. It continues throughout adult life.

COMMUNICATIVE COMPETENCE - The speaker's ability to effectively communicate an intentional message so as to alter the listener's attitudes, beliefs, and/or behaviors (Lucas, 1980).

COMMUNICATION UNIT - A group of words that cannot be further divided without the loss of their essential meaning (Loban, 1976). It can also be defined as each independent clause with its modifier.

COMMUNICATIVE DISORDERS - An impairment in the ability to: receive and/or process a symbol system; represent concepts or symbol systems; and/or transmit and use symbol systems. The impairment is observed in disorders of hearing, language, and/or speech processes (ASHA, 1982).

CONCEPT - A grouping of objects on the basis of some common attribute, relationship, or characteristic. A concept represents the attributes common to several different events. Concepts are means by which students organize experiences.

CONSERVATION - The recognition that one aspect of something can remain the same (e.g., volume) while another aspect is altered (e.g., width of container).

CONVERSATIONAL PARTNER - One member of a dyad.

CONVERSATIONAL UNIT - The utterance(s) of one conversational partner that continue(s) until the other conversational partner initiates an independent utterance.

COPULA VERB - A form of the be verb which joins a subject to its predicate and functions as the primary verb in the sentence (contrast with auxiliary verb). Copula verbs include: seem, appear, feel, remain, become.

CRITERION-REFERENCED TEST - A student's development of certain skills assessed in terms of absolute levels of mastery. Criterion-referenced tests are objective and arranged in a hierarchical order of sequential skills. Ratio scores are obtained (e.g., the students identify the main idea of the speaker three out of four times).

DEDUCTIVE REASONING - Reasoning from the general to the specific.

DEIXIS - Social interchange facilitating language acquisition through sharing the reciprocal roles of speaker and hearer (Lucas, 1980).

DEPENDENT CLAUSE - Equivalent to a subordinate clause, it acts as a subject, complement, or modifier, but has a subject or verb of its own. It is fully introduced by a subordinating word that is stated or understood (e.g., that, which).

DEVELOPMENTAL LANGUAGE DISORDER - A disorder in language which occurs during the developmental period between birth and age 22 years.

DISTINCTIVE FEATURES - Attributes that are required to differentiate one phoneme from another in a language including the presence or absence of voicing and contrasts in the various manners of articulation.

EXPRESSIVE LANGUAGE - Production of language for the purpose of communication. Speaking and writing are considered expressive language skills.

EXTRAPOLATION - A process of estimating the scores of a test beyond the range of available data (Compton, 1980).

FIGURATIVE LANGUAGE - Informal usage of language including slang and idiomatic expressions.

FILLED PAUSE - Any pause during which the speaker emits sounds such as "er," "um," "ah" to initiate or maintain an utterance, or emits verbal mazes, confused and tangled use of words characterized by false starts, hesitations, and meaningless repetition of words.

FRAGMENT - Any utterance that is not a sentence.

GESTURES

> SUPPORTIVE GESTURES - Movements of the hands/arms, shoulders, or head that aid (assist) in the communication of the verbal message during the conversational unit.

> NONSUPPORTIVE GESTURES - Movements of the hands/arms, shoulders, or head which do not aid (assist) in the communication of the verbal message during the conversational unit.

GRAMMAR - The accurate and appropriate application of morphological and syntactical rules of the language.

HYPOTHETICAL-DEDUCTIVE THINKING - Thinking which involves considering all possibilities and experimenting (hypothesizing) from that point.

ILLOCUTIONARY ACTS - Uttering sounds or symbols said to have meaning in the speaker's intentions and in a subsequent effect on the hearer (Lucas, 1980).

INDEPENDENT CLAUSE - Equivalent to a main clause, it contains a subject and verb, and expresses a complete thought. It can stand alone as a grammatical sentence.

INDEPENDENT UTTERANCE - Any nonsimultaneous vocalization.

INDUCTIVE REASONING - Reasoning from the specific to the general.

INITIATION - Onset of vocalization.

INTELLIGENCE - A global concept composed of factors such as cognitive skills, abstract verbal and numerical processing, memory, and the ability to learn, solve problems, and engage in reasoning.

INTELLIGENCE QUOTIENT (IQ) - An expression of a student's mental ability as determined by performance on an intelligence test. Many tests used to establish IQ rely upon the student's current knowledge of the world, rather than on the student's potential to acquire knowledge. A student with a mental age equal to chronological age would have an IQ score of 100.

INTERPOLATION - A process of estimating an intermediate value between two known points (Compton, 1980). For example, if a raw score of 62 is equivalent to a grade norm of 4.0, and a raw score of 60 is equivalent to a grade norm of 3.8, then one can interpolate that a raw score of 61 would be equivalent to a grade norm of 3.9.

INTERRUPTION - Any vocalization or gesture made by one conversational partner during the turn of the other conversational partner.

VERBAL:

POSITIVE - Any affirmative vocalization
NEGATIVE - Any nonaffirmative vocalization

NONVERBAL:

POSITIVE - Any affirmative head/facial/body movement
NEGATIVE - Any nonaffirmative head/facial/body movement

LANGUAGE - Language is a complex and dynamic system of conventional symbols that is used in various modes for thought and communication.

Contemporary views of human language hold that:

-- Language evolves within specific historical, social, and cultural context

-- Language, as rule governed behavior, is described by at least five parameters -- phonologic, morphologic, syntactic, semantic, and pragmatic

-- Language learning and use are determined by the interaction of biological, cognitive, psychosocial, and environmental factors

223

-- Effective use of language for communication requires a broad understanding of human interaction including such associated factors as nonverbal cues, motivation, and sociocultural roles

LANGUAGE DIFFERENCE - A person meets the norms of his/her primary linguistic community but does not meet the norms of standard English (ASHA, LC-20, Nov. 1982).

LANGUAGE DISORDER - The impairment or deviant development of comprehension and/or use of a spoken, written, and/or other symbol system. The disorder may involve form, content, and/or function of language (ASHA, 1982).

LINGUISTIC - The scientific study of language, its form and function.

MAZE - A series of words or unattached fragments which do not constitute a communication unit and are not necessary to the communication unit (Loban, 1976).

MEAN (M) - Given a set of scores, it is the average of those scores (i.e., sum of all scores divided by the number of scores).

MEDIAN (MD) - Given a set of ranked scores, it is the middle point. The same number of scores fall above the median as fall below it in a distribution.

MODAL VERBS - A subcategory of auxiliary verbs that includes words like can, could, may, might, will, would, must, shall, should.

MODE (MO) - Given a set of scores, it is the score that occurs most frequently.

MORPHEME - The smallest unit of speech that has meaning. Morphemes may be bound (e.g., "ing" used with present progressive verbs) or free (e.g., any word not having a bound morpheme, such as "man," "dog").

MORPHOLOGY - The linguistic rule system that governs the structure of words and the construction of word forms from the basic elements of meaning (ASHA, 1982).

NEGATION - The appearance of a negative word or phrase in a sentence.

DOUBLE NEGATION - The appearance of two words that denote negation within the same sentence.

NONSPECIFIC LANGUAGE - Language with low information content, including indefinite pronouns (e.g., they, them) and nouns such as "this," "thing," "something," "nothing" with no discernible referent point established.

NORM-REFERENCED TESTS - A test that has undergone standardization procedures. A student's performance can be compared to other students who are the same chronological age. All norm-referenced tests are standardized tests.

OPERATION - The mental process of thinking about several aspects of a concept simultaneously; an understanding of the relationship among concepts.

PASSIVE VOICE - The subject of a sentence is receiving an action (e.g., The puppy is being saved by the girl.).

PERCENTILE RANK - A type of converted score that expresses a student's score relative to his/her group in percentile points (Compton, 1980). A percentile rank indicates the percentage of students tested who have scored equal to or lower than a specific score. For example, a percentile rank of 80 (corresponding to a score of 70) means that 80% of the students who took the test had a score of 70 or less than 70.

PERLOCUTIONARY ACTS - The effects of specific acts on a hearer (Lucas, 1980).

PHONEME - The smallest unit of sound in a language, not possessing meaning. There are many more phonemes in the English language than there are letters in the alphabet.

PHONOLOGY - The sound system of a language and the linguistic rules that govern the sound combinations (ASHA, 1982).

PRAGMATICS - The sociolinguistic system that patterns the use of language in communication which may be expressed motorically, vocally, and verbally (ASHA, 1982).

PROPORTIONALITY - The relationship between two or more ratios.

QUESTION - A sentence in an interrogative form.

> INTERROGATIVE REVERSAL - Sentence in which the subject and the verb phrase, or part thereof, are transposed.

> TAG - "Yes-no" questions formulated by making a sentence followed immediately, within the same sentence, by a confirmatory comment such as "didn't you," "wasn't it," etc.

> RISING INTONATION - "Yes-no" questions formulated by saying a sentence in which the last several words are upwardly inflected.

225

WH - Questions which are characterized by the presence of a "Wh" marker (i.e., what, who, whom, whose, when, why, how).

RATE OF SPEECH - The number of words per minute at which the speaker converses.

RECEPTIVE LANGUAGE - Comprehension or understanding of language. Listening and reading are considered receptive language skills.

REGISTER - The range of word and sentence choices and language styles available to a speaker (Wiig and Semel, 1980).

RELIABILITY - The stability or consistency of test scores. If a test is highly reliable, the student would receive the same score if it were readministered (assuming no changes had occurred).

SENTENCE - The unit of linguistic measurement.

SIMPLE - A sentence which has one noun phrase and one verb phrase in a subject-predicate relationship.

COMPLEX - A sentence which contains more than one noun phrase and/or verb phrase and is characterized by the presence of a coordinating or subordinating conjunction and/or an embedded clause.

SEMANTICS - The psycholinguistic system that patterns the content of an utterance, intent, and meaning of words and sentences (ASHA, 1982).

SERIATION - The operation of ordering objects or events (e.g., small to large).

SPEECH - A motor behavior or act of respiration, phonation, articulation, and resonation.

STANDARD DEVIATION (SD) - The extent of deviation of the distribution of scores from the Mean. A common measurement of variation. About 68% of the scores lie within one standard deviation below or above the Mean in a normal distribution.

STANDARDIZATION - The process of administering a test to a group of students to determine uniform or standard procedures and methods of interpretation.

STANDARDIZED TEST - A test that has undergone standardization and provides data on validity and reliability. Items are empirically selected and specific directions for administration, scoring, and interpretation are provided.

STRATEGY - Learning strategies are defined as techniques, principles, or rules that will facilitate the acquisition, manipulation, integration, storage, and retrieval of information
across situations and settings (Alley and Deshler, 1979).

SYNTAX - The linguistic rule governing the order and combination
of words to form sentences and the relationships among the
elements within a sentence (ASHA, 1982).

TOPIC SHIFT - Any shift from the current topic of discussion.

ABRUPT - Any topic shift that was made quickly and had no
immediate referent.

GRADUAL - Any topic shift that had one or more transitional
utterances that connected the immediate topic and the one
which followed.

TURN NUMBER - The number of speaking turns of one member of the
dyad.

TURN SHIFT - A new conversational unit.

TURN TIME - The sum of the durations (amount of time) of one conversational partner's speaking turns.

UTTERANCE - Any vocalization.

VALIDITY - The extent to which a test measures what it is designed to measure (Compton, 1980). There are several types
of validity:

CONTENT VALIDITY - The content of a test samples a specific
subject matter. Content validity concerns how well the content of the test samples the behavior domain about which
conclusions are to be made. Achievement tests are mostly
concerned with this kind of validity.

FACE VALIDITY - A test is assumed to be valid simply by
definition (e.g., a scale is a valid instrument to measure
weight). Face validity is the idea that the test is valid.

PREDICTED VALIDITY - Predictions about students are often
made on the basis of test scores. Predictive validity concerns how effective these predictions were as substantiated
by data obtained at a later time (e.g., the correlation of
IQ scores with school grades).

WORD RETRIEVAL - The ability to recall words as needed for normal
verbal communication.

BIBLIOGRAPHY

BIBLIOGRAPHY

Allen, R. & Brown, K. Developing communication competence in children. Skokie, IL: National Textbook Company, 1976.

Alley, G. & Deshler, D. Teaching the learning disabled adolescent: Strategies and methods. Denver, CO: Love Publishing Co., 1979.

Alson, L. & Swidler, A. A pilot program for language development in the educable adolescent. Language, Speech, and Hearing Services in Schools, April 1976, 7(2), 102-105.

Aram, D. & Nation, J. Preschool language disorders and subsequent language and academic difficulties. Journal of Communication Disorders, 1980, 13, 159-170.

Arizona Department of Education. Communication skills chart - speaking/writing and Communication skills chart - listening/reading. Tempe, AZ: Department of Education, 1980.

Arlin, P. Cognitive development in adulthood: A fifth stage? Developmental Psychology, September 1979, 11, 602-606.

Auslin, Myra Shulman, Hold your horses, a workbook of idioms. Beaverton, OR: Dormac, Inc., 1979.

Avery, A., Rider, K., & Haynes-Clements, L. Communication skills training for adolescents: A five month follow-up. Adolescence, Summer 1982, 16(62).

Backlund, P., Booth, J., Moore, M., Parks, A., & Van Rheenen, D. A national survey of state practices in speaking and listening skill assessment. Communication Education, April 1982, 31.

Backlund, P., Brown, K., Gurry, J., & Jandt, F. Recommendations for assessing speaking and listening skills. Communication Education, January 1982, 31.

Baggett, L. Behavior that communicates understanding as evaluated by teen-agers. Paper presented at the American Personnel and Guidance Association Convention, Las Vegas, Nevada, March 1969.

Baken, D. Adolescence in America from idea to social fact. In: Wincler, A.E. (Ed.); Adolescence: Contemporary studies (2nd Ed). New York: D. Van Nostrand Co., 1974.

Baker, H.J. & Leland, B. Detroit tests of learning aptitude. Indianapolis, IN: Bobbs-Merrill Co., 1967.

Bassett, R., Whittington, N., & Staton-Spicer, A. The basics in speaking and listening for high school graduates: What should be assessed? Communication Education, November 1978, 27, 293-303.

Bender, M. & Valletutti, P. Teaching functional academics: A curriculum guide for adolescents and adults with learning problems. Baltimore, MD: University Park Press, 1982.

Benedict, R. Continuities and discontinuities in cultural conditioning. In: Skolnik, A. (Ed.) Rethinking childhood: Perspectives on development and society. Boston, MA: Little, Brown and Company, 1976.

Bernstein, B. Elaborated and restricted codes: Their social origins and some consequences. American Anthropologist, 1964, 66, 55-69.

Bloom, B.S. (Ed.) Taxonomy of educational objectives: The classification of educational goals: Handbook I: Cognitive domain. New York: Longman, Inc., 1956.

Bloom, B.S., Hastings, J.T., & Modaus, G.F. Handbook of formative and summative evaluation of student learning. New York: McGraw-Hill Book Company, 1971.

Bloom, L., & Lahey, M. Language development and language disorders. New York: John Wiley and Sons, 1978.

Boehm, A. Boehm test of basic concepts. New York, New York: The Psychological Corporation, 1971.

Botel, M. Botel reading inventory. Chicago, IL: Follett Educational Corp., 1970.

Boyce, N., Godwin, E., & Larson, V. Communicative disorders services: Grades 7-12. Unpublished survey, Eau Claire, WI: University of Wisconsin-Eau Claire, Dept. of Communication Disorders, 1979.

Brigance, A. Inventory of basic skills. North Billerica, MA: Curriculum Associates, Inc., 1981.

Brigance, A. Inventory of essential skills. North Billerica, MA: Curriculum Associates, Inc., 1981.

Broughton, J. Beyond formal operations: Theoretical thoughts in adolescence. Teacher's College Records, September 1977, 79, 87-97.

Brown, J.I. & Carlsen, G.R. Brown-Carlsen listening comprehension test. New York: Harcourt, Brace and World, Inc., 1955.

Brown, V. Curriculum development resources. In: Mann, Goodman, and Wiederholt (Eds.), Teaching the learning disabled adolescent. Boston, MA: Houghton Mifflin Company, 1978.

Brubaker, S. Workbook for aphasia. Detroit, MI: Wayne State University Press, 1978.

Bruininks, V.L. Designing instructional activities for students with language/learning disabilities. Language Arts, February 1978, 55(2).

Burns, M. Book of think ("or how to solve a problem twice your size"). Boston, MA: Little, Brown & Co., 1976.

Castello, R. Listening guide - a first step toward note-taking and listening skills. Journal of Reading, 1976, 19, 289-290.

Chapman, R. Pragmatic development. Paper presented at Wisconsin Speech and Hearing Association, Madison, Wisconsin, April 28, 1979.

Chappell, G. Oral language performance of upper elementary school students obtained via story reformulation. Language, Speech, and Hearing Services in Schools. October 1980, 4, 236-250.

Chappell, G. A cognitive-linguistic intervention program: Basic concept formation level. Language, Speech, and Hearing Services in Schools, January 1977, 8(1), 23-32.

Choose your own adventure series. New York, NY: Bantam Books, Harper and Row Publishers, Inc., 1978.

Classification and organization skills - developmental. North Billerica, MA: Curriculum Associates, Inc., 1981.

Cognitive-language-communication assessment instrument. Schofield, WI: D.C. Everest Public Schools. Revised, 1981.

Cohen, A. The influence of friendship on children's communication. Journal of Social Psychology, 1980, 112(2), 207-213.

Compensatory education in early adolescence. Menlo Park, CA: Stanford Research Institute, 1974.

Compton, C. A guide to 65 tests for special education. Belmont, CA: Pitman Learning, Inc., 1980.

Conger, J.J. Adolescence and youth: Psychological development in a changing world. New York: Harper and Row, 1973.

Copeland, R. Diagnostic and learning activities in mathematics for children. New York, NY: Macmillan Publishing Co., Inc., 1974.

230

Costanzo, P. & Shaw, M.   Conformity of a function of age level. *Child Development*, December 1966, 37, 967-75.

Crager, R. *Test of concept utilization*. Los Angeles, CA: Western Psychological Services, 1972.

Cunningham, P.M. & Cunningham, J.W. Improving listening in content area subjects. *National Association of Secondary School Board Principals*, 1976, 60, 26-31.

Curriculum guide: Speech-language program, secondary level. Schofield, WI: D.C. Everest Public Schools, 1980.

Darley, F.L. (Ed.) *Evaluation of appraisal techniques in speech and language pathology*. Reading, MA: Addison-Wesley Publishing Co., 1979.

Dickson, W.P. & Patterson, J. Evaluating referential communication games for teaching speaking and listening skills. *Communication Education*. January 1981, 30.

DiVesta, F. & Gray, G.S. Listening and note-taking, *Journal of Educational Psychology*, 1972, 63, 8-14.

Dolch, E. *Basic sight vocabulary cards*. Champaign, IL: Garrard Publishing Co., 1949.

Doll, E. *Vineland Social Maturity Scale*. Circle Pines, MN: American Guidance Service, Inc., 1965.

Dorval, B. *The development of conversation*. Paper presented at the Biennial Southeastern Conference on Human Development "6th," Alexandria, VA, April 1980.

Duker, S. *Listening readings, vol. 2*. Metuchen, NJ: The Scarecrow Press, Inc., 1971.

Dunn, L. *Peabody picture vocabulary test - revised*. Circle Pines, MN: American Guidance Service, 1980.

Durrell, D.D. *Durrell analysis of reading difficulty*. New York: Harcourt, Brace, Jovanovich, 1955.

Duska, D. & Wheelan, M. *Moral development: A guide to Piaget and Kohlberg*. New York: Paulist Press, 1975.

Effective listening: Listener's response book. New York: Xerox Corporation, 1967.

Eggleston, P. & Riggs, R. *Listening skills development*. Redmond, OR: The Oregon Teaching Center, 1982.

Eisenson, J. *Examining for aphasia (rev. ed.)*. New York: Psychological Corp., 1954.

Elkind, D. Recent research on cognitive development in adolescents. In: Sigmund, E., Dragastin, S. & Elder, G., Jr. (Eds.) Adolescence in the life cycle: Psychological change and social context. New York: John Wiley, 1975.

Elkind, D. Quantity conception in junior and senior high school students. Child Development, September 1961, 32, 551-560.

Emerick, L. The parent interview. Danville, IL: Interstate Printers and Publishers, Inc., 1969.

Emerick, L. & Hatten, J. Diagnosis and evaluation in speech pathology (2nd ed.). Englewood Cliffs, NJ: Prentice-Hall Inc., 1979.

Ennis, R.H. Critical thinking readiness in grades 1-12. Ithaca, NY: Cornell University, 1965.

Erikson, E. Identity: Youth and crisis. New York: W.W. Norton, 1968.

Faix, T.L. Listening as a human relations art. Elementary English, 1975, 52, 409-426.

Feuerstein, R. The dynamic assessment of retarded performers. Baltimore, MD: University Park Press, 1979.

Feuerstein, R. Instrumental enrichment. Baltimore, MD: University Park Press, 1980.

Fiester, A.R. & Giambra, L.M. Language indices of vocational success in mentally retarded adults, American Journal of Mental Deficiency, 1972, 77, 332-337.

Fleishman, A. Sense and nonsense, a study in human communication. San Francisco, CA: International Society of General Semantics, 1971.

Fleishman, A. Troubled talk! San Francisco, CA: International Society of General Semantics, 1973.

Flynn, J. Curriculum adaptation for learning-disabled adolescents. Paper presented at Comprehensive Child Care Center Conference, Gunderson Clinic, La Crosse, WI, May 1982.

French, R. Nonverbal patterns in youth culture. Educational Leadership, April 1978, 541-546.

Freud, S. The ego and the mechanism of defense. New York: International Universities Press, 1948.

Furth, H. Piaget for teachers. Englewood Cliffs, NJ: Prentice-Hall, Inc., 1970.

Furth, H. & Wachs, H. Piaget's theory in practice, thinking goes to school. Fair Lawn, NJ: Oxford University Press, Inc., 1974.

Gates, A.I. & McKillop, A.S. Gates-McKillop reading diagnostic tests. New York: Teacher's College Press, Columbia University, 1962.

Gilligan, C. New map of development: New vision of maturity. American Journal of Orthopsychiatry, April 1982, 52(2), 199-212.

Ginsburg, H. & Opper, S. Piaget's theory of intellectual development. New Jersey: Prentice-Hall, Inc., 1969.

Gleser, G., Winget, C. & Seligman, R. Content scaling of affect in adolescent speech sample. Journal of Youth and Adolescence, 1979, 8(3), 283-297.

Gorman, R.M. Discovering Piaget: A guide for teachers. Columbus, OH: Charles E. Merrill Publishing Company, 1972.

Greenes, C., Gregory, J. & Seymour, D. Successful problem solving techniques. Palo Alto, CA: Creative Publications, Inc., 1977.

Grice, H.P. Logic and conversation. In: Cole, P. & Morgan, J.L. (Eds.), Syntax and semantics: vol. 3, speech acts. New York: Academic Press, 1975.

Gruenewald, L. & Pollak, S. Analyzing language interactions in academics. Journal of Learning Disabilities, 1975, 8, 544-550.

Hall, M. Teaching reading as a language experience. Columbus, OH: Charles E. Merrill Publishing Company, 1976.

Hall, S. Adolescence: Its psychology and its relations to physiology, anthropology, sociology, sex, crime, religion, and education. New York: Appleton Press, 1904.

Halliday, M.A.K. Learning how to mean: Explorations in the development of language. New York: Elsevior North Holland Publishing Co., 1975.

Hammill, D.D., Brown, V.L., Larsen, S.C. & Wiederholt, J.L. Test of adolescent language: A multi-dimensional approach to assessment (TOAL). East Aurora, NY: Slosson Educational Publications, Inc., 1980.

Harnadek, A. Mind benders. Troy, MI: Midwest Publications Co., Inc., 1978.

Harnadek, A. Basic thinking skills. Troy, MI: Midwest Publications Co., Inc., 1977.

Harnadek, A. <u>Critical thinking, book 1</u>. Troy, MI: Midwest Publications Co., Inc., 1976.

Harnishfeger, L. <u>Basic practice in listening</u>. Denver, CO: Love Publishing Co., 1977.

<u>Harry Stottlemeier's discovery</u>. Institute for the Advancement of Philosophy for Children. Montclair State College, Upper Montclair, NJ, 1974.

Horn, E. The curriculum for the gifted. Some principles and an illustration. <u>Twenty-third Yearbook of the National Society for the Study of Education</u>. Bloomington, IL: Public School Publishing Co., 1924.

Hymes, D. Competence and performance in linguistic theory. In: Huxley, R. & Ingram, E. (Eds.) <u>Language acquisition: Models and methods</u>. New York: Academic Press, 1971.

Inhelder, B. & Piaget, J. <u>The growth of logical thinking from childhood to adolescence - an essay on the construction of formal operational structures</u>. Translated by Parson, A. & Milgram, S., New York: Basic Books, 1958.

Insel, E. & Edson, A. <u>Reading listening comprehension - level IV</u>. Freeport, NY: Educational Activities, 1976.

Insel, E. & Edson, A. <u>Reading vocabulary development creature features</u>. Freeport, NY: Educational Activities, Inc., 1979.

James, G., Whitley, C.G. & Bode, S. <u>Listening in and speaking out: Intermediate</u>. New York: Longman, Inc., 1980.

Johnson, D. <u>Language/learning disabilities in young adults</u>. Paper presented at American Speech-Language-Hearing Association, North Central Regional Conference, Milwaukee, WI, August 1982.

Johnson, I.M. <u>Developing the listening skills</u>. Baldwin, NY: Educational Activities, Inc., 1974.

Johnson, R., et al. <u>Childrens' ability to recognize and improve upon socially inept communications</u>. Paper presented at the Annual Convention of American Psychologists Association (88th), Montreal, Quebec, Canada, September 1980.

Jorgensen, C., Barrett, M., Huisingh, R. & Zachman, L. <u>The Word Test</u>. Moline, IL: LinguiSystems, 1981.

Kagan, J.A. A conception of early adolescence. <u>Daeclalus</u>, Fall 1971, 997-1012.

Kellman, M., Flood, C. & Yoder, D. <u>Language assessment tasks</u>. New Holstein, WI. Rev. 1978.

King, R., Jones, C. & Lasky, E. In retrospect: A fifteen-year follow-up report of speech-language-disordered children. Language, Speech, and Hearing Services in Schools, January 1982, 13(1), 24-32.

Kirk, S.A., McCarthy, J.J. & Kirk, W.D. Illinois test of psycholinguistic ability (rev. ed.) Urbana, IL: University of Illinois Press, 1968.

Klein, M., Pasch, M. & Frew, T. Curriculum analysis and design for retarded learners. Columbus, OH: Charles E. Merrill Publishing Co., 1979.

Knowles, M. The adult learner: A neglected species. Houston, TX: Gulf Publishing Company, 1973.

Kohlberg, L. The cognitive-developmental approach to moral education. Phi Delta Kappa, 1975, 36-51.

Kretschmer, R., Jr., & Kretschmer, L. Perspectives in audiology series: Language development and intervention with the hearing impaired. Baltimore, MD: University Park Press, 1978.

Labinowicz, E. The Piaget primer. Menlo Park, CA: Addison-Wesley Publishing Company, 1980.

Larson, V. & Boyce, N. ABC's: Adolescents' behavior in conversation (in preparation).

Lawson, A. & Wollman, W. Encouraging the transition from concrete to formal cognitive functioning - an experiment. Journal of Research in Science Teaching, September 1976, 413-430.

Lazzari, A. & Peters, P. HELP: Handbook of exercises for language processing - vol. 1. Moline, IL: LinguiSystems, Inc., 1981.

Lazzari, A. & Peters, P. HELP: Handbook of exercises for language processing - vol. 2. Moline, IL: LinguiSystems, Inc., 1981.

Legislative Council Resolution 20, American Speech-Language-Hearing Association Convention, Toronto, Ontario, Canada, November 1982.

Let's look at logic. Guidance Associates, New York: Harcourt, Brace, Jovanovich, Inc., 1977.

Lewis, T. & Nichols, R. Speaking and listening: A guide to effective oral-aural communication. Dubuque, IA: William C. Brown, 1965.

Lipman, M. Philosophy for children. Meta-Philosophy, January 1976, 7(1), 17-39.

Lipman, M. & Sharp, A.M. Harry Stottlemeier's discovery. Upper Montclair, NJ: Institute for the Advancement of Philosophy for Children, 1974.

Loban, W. Language development: Kindergarten through grade 12. Urbana, IL: National Council of Teachers of English, 1976.

Longhurst, T. & Siegel, G. Effects of communication failure on speaker and listener behavior. Journal of Speech and Hearing Research, 1973, 16, 128-140.

Lozano, F. & Sturtevant, J. Lifestyles. New York: Longman, Inc., 1981.

Lucas, E. Semantic and pragmatic language disorders: Assessment and remediation. Rockville, MD: Aspen Systems Corp., 1980.

Lundsteen, S. Listening: Its impact on reading and the other language arts. IL: NCTE/ERIC, 1971.

Lewis, S. & Rosenblum, L. (Eds.) Interaction, conversation, and the development of language. New York: John Wiley and Sons, Inc., 1977.

MacWhinney, B. & Bates, E. Sentential devices for conveying giveness and newness: A cross-cultural developmental study. Journal of Verbal Learning and Verbal Behavior, 1978, 17, 539-558.

Mahoney, D. Survival skills from the classroom. Perspective for Teachers of the Hearing Impaired, September 1982, 1(1), 11-13.

Markgraf, B. An observational study determining the amount of time that students in the 10th and 12th grades are expected to listen in the classroom in listening readings. Ducar, S. (Ed.), New York: Scarecrow Press, 1966.

Marshall, E. Attribute games: Problem solving and reasoning skills development. Boston, MA: Teaching Resources, 1971.

Martorano, S. A developmental analysis of performance on Piaget's formal operation tasks. Developmental Psychology, 1977, 13(6), 666-672.

McCroskey, J., Andersen, J., Richmond, V. & Wheeless, L. Communication apprehension of elementary and secondary students and teachers. Communication Education, April 1981, 30.

McLeod, A.M., Listening, writing and the realm of imagination. Clearing House, 1979, 53, 8-10.

McNeil, M.R. & Prescott, T. Revised token test. Baltimore, Maryland: University Park Press, 1978.

236

Mead, M. _Coming of age in Samoa_. New York: New American Library, 1950.

Meeker, M. _The structure of intellect, its interpretation and uses_. Columbus, OH: Charles E. Merrill Publishing Co., 1969.

Meeker, M. & Meeker, R. _SOI learning abilities test_. El Segundo, CA: SOI Institute, 1975.

Menyuk, P. _Language and maturization_. Cambridge, MA: MIT Press, 1978.

Miller, J. _Assessing language production in children_. Baltimore, MD: University Park Press, 1981.

Miller, J. & Yoder, D. _Grammatical comprehension test_. Madison, WI: University of Wisconsin, 1973 (out of print).

Miller, S. & Judd, W. _Thinkerthings: A student generated approach to language experience_. Menlo Park, CA: Addison-Wesley Publishing Company, 1975.

Minnesota Department of Education. _Some essential learner outcomes in communications/language arts_. (Curriculum Bulletin No. 61). St. Paul, MN: Department of Education, 1982.

Morehead, D.M. & Ingram, D. The development of base syntax in normal and linguistically deviant children. _Journal of Speech and Hearing Research_, 1973, 16, 330-352.

Morgansteen, S. & Smith, M.C. _Thematic language stimulation: A workbook for aphasics and their clinicians_. Tucson, AZ: Communication Skill Builders, 1982.

Morley, J. _Improving aural comprehension_. Ann Arbor, MI: The University of Michigan Press, 1972.

Morris, K. & Cinnamon, K. _A handbook of verbal group exercises_. St. Louis, MO: APP Skills Press, CMA Publications, 1974.

Mueller, P. _Suggested modal pitch level and range by age and sex_. Personal Communication, University of Wisconsin-Eau Claire, October, 1982.

Mullica, K. _Sentence solitaire_. Tucson, AZ: Communication Skill Builders, 1982.

Myers, R.E. Rediscovering listening: It's basic and it's free. _Clearing House_, 1979, 53, 183-185.

National Youth Workers Conference, in Washington, D.C., Personal Communication, July 1982.

Neimark, E. Current status of formal operations research. <u>Human Development</u>, 1979, 22, 60-67.

Neville, M.A. Listening is an art: Practice it. <u>Elementary English</u>, 1959, 36, 226+.

Nicolosi, L., Harryman, E. & Kresheck, J. <u>Terminology of communication disorders, speech, language, hearing</u>. Baltimore, MD: The Williams and Wilkins Company, 1978.

Oklahoma Project. <u>Exceptions: A handbook for teachers of mainstream students</u>. Project Mainstream in Cooperation with the Oklahoma Child Service Demonstration Center and Developer/ Demonstrator Project, Learning Disabilities Programs, Cushing, OK, 1982.

Oller, J., Jr. <u>Language testing at school</u>. London, England: Longman Group, Ltd., 1979.

<u>Oral proficiency program, secondary schools</u>. Gary, IN: Gary Community School Corporation, 1977.

<u>Oregon Trail</u>. Minnesota Educational Computer Consortium, St. Paul, MN, 1980.

Oyer, H. <u>Auditory communication for the hard of hearing</u>. Englewood Cliffs, NJ: Prentice-Hall, Inc., 1966.

Peets, R., et al. Chair - Committee on Language, Speech, and Hearing Services in the Schools. Definitions - communicative disorders and variations. <u>American Speech-Language-Hearing Association</u>, November 1982, 24(11), 949-950.

Phillips, J.L. <u>The origins of intellect: Piaget's theory</u>. San Francisco, CA: H. Freemond and Co., 1969.

Pirie, J. & Pirie, A. <u>Thirty lessons on note-taking</u>. North Billerica, MA: Curriculum Associates, Inc., 1976.

Poole, M. Social class, sex and linguistic coding. <u>Lang. Speech</u>, 1979, 22(1), 49-68.

Poole, M. A comparison of oral and written code elaborations. <u>Lang. Speech</u>, 1976, 19(4), 305-312.

Potter, R. <u>Making sense: Exploring semantics and critical thinking</u>. New York, NY: Globe Book Co., Inc., 1974.

Prather, E., Brenner, A. & Hughes, K. A mini-screening language test for adolescents. <u>Language-Speech-Hearing Services in Schools</u>, April 1981, 12(2), 67-73.

Prather, E., Beecher, S., Stafford, M. & Wallace, E. Screening test of adolescent language. Seattle, WA: University of Washington Press, 1980.

Problem solving: Using your head creatively. Pleasantville, NY: Human Relations Media, 1978.

A program to improve listening. Washington, DC: National Education Association of the United States, 1964.

Project Stile. Learning how to learn: Methods, objectives, activities for teaching learning strategies for learning disabled adolescents. Lawrence, KS: Lawrence High School, 1979.

Rankin, R. The measurement of the ability to understand spoken language. Unpublished dissertation. University of Michigan, 1926.

Rees, N. & Wollner, S. A Taxonomy of Pragmatic Abilities. Educational Telephone Network Conference, February 1982.

Rees, N.S. & Shulman, M. I don't understand what you mean by comprehension. Journal of Speech and Hearing Disorders, May 1978, 43(2), 208-219.

Rice, F.P. The adolescent: Development, relationships and culture. Boston, MA: Allyn and Bacon, Inc., 1975.

Richey, J. Survival vocabularies. Hayward, CA: Jannus Book Publishers, 1978.

Richey, J. Sign language: A survival vocabulary. Hayward, CA: Jannus Book Publishers, 1977.

Ritter, E. The social-cognitive development of adolescents: Implications for the teaching of speech. Communication Education, 1981, 30.

Ritter, E. Social perspective taking ability, cognitive complexity and listener adapted communication in early and late adolescence, Communication Monograph, March 1979, 46, 40-51.

Ross, C. Cognitive challenge cards. Novato, CA: Academic Therapy Publications, 1978.

Ruben, B.D. & Budd, R.W. Human communication handbook: Simulations and games, vol. 1. Rochelle Park, NJ: Hayden Book Company, Inc., 1975.

Ruben, B. Human communication handbook: Simulations and games, vol. 2. Rochelle Park, NJ: Hayden Book Co., Inc., 1978.

Rubin, R. Communication competency assessment instrument. Annandale, VA: Speech Communication Association, 1982.

Rubin, R. Assessing speaking and listening competence at the college level: The communication competency assessment instrument, Communication Education, January 1982, 31, 19-32.

Sabun, D. Communications: The transfer of meaning. Beverly Hills, CA: Glencoe Press, 1968.

Searle, J. A classification of illocutionary acts. Language Soc., 1976, 5, 123.

Semel, E.M. & Wiig, E.M. Clinical evaluation of language functions. Columbus, OH: Charles E. Merrill Publishing Co., 1980.

Sequential tests of educational progress (STEP) - Listening. Princeton, NJ: Educational Testing Service, 1958.

Siegal, M. Kohlberg versus Piaget: To what extent has one theory eclipsed the other? Merrill-Palmer Quarterly, October 1980, 26(4), 285-297.

Sigel, I. & Cocking, R. Cognitive development from childhood to adolescence - A constructivist perspective. New York: Holt, Rinehart & Winston, 1977.

Simon, C. Communication therapy: After is-verbing, then what? Paper presented at American Speech-Language-Hearing Association Convention in Los Angeles, CA, November 1981.

Simon, C. Communicative competency: A functional-pragmatic language program. Tucson, AZ: Communication Skill Builders, Inc., 1980.

Simon, C.S. Communicative competence: A functional-pragmatic approach to language therapy. Tucson, AZ: Communication Skill Builders, Inc., 1979.

Survival guides. Hayward, CA: Jannus Book Publishers, 1977.

Tanner, J. Growth at adolescence, Second Ed. Oxford: Blackwell Scientific Publications, Ltd., 1962.

Tobias, J. A glossary of affluent suburban juvenile slanguage. Adolescence, Spring 1980, 15(57), 227-230.

Tutolo, D. Teaching critical listening. Language Arts, 1975, 52, 1108-1112.

Utah State Board of Education. Functional competencies required for high school graduation: Teacher handbook. Salt Lake City, UT: State Board of Education, 1978.

Valletutti, P. & Bender, M. _Teaching interpersonal and community living skills: A curriculum model for handicapped adolescents and adults_. Baltimore, MD: University Park Press, 1982.

Vermont Dept. of Education. _Basic competencies: Teacher's guide for basic competencies in reasoning_. Montpelier, VT: State Dept. of Education, 1979.

Vermont Dept. of Education. _Basic competencies: A manual of information and guidelines for teachers and administrators_. Montpelier, VT: State Dept. of Education, March 1977.

Wadsworth, B.J. _Piaget for the classroom teacher_. New York: Longman Publishing Co., 1978.

Watkins, B. Demand grows for reforming high schools. _Chronicle of Higher Education_. November 1982.

Weber, K. _Thinklab_. Toronto, Ontario, Canada: Science Research Associates, 1974.

Werner, E. A study of communication time. _Masters Thesis_, University of Maryland, College Park, MD, 1975.

Wiig, E. _Let's talk: Developing prosocial communication skills_. Columbus, OH: Charles E. Merrill Publishing Co., 1982.

Wiig, E. _Let's talk inventory for adolescents_. Columbus, OH: Charles E. Merrill Publishing Co., 1982.

Wiig, E. _Identifying language disorders in adolescents_. Oral presentation at Gunderson Clinic, La Crosse, WI, May 1982.

Wiig, E. & Harris, S. Perception and interpretation of nonverbally expressed emotions by adolescents with learning disabilities. _Perceptual and motor skills, vol. 38_, 1974, 38, 239-245.

Wiig, E.H. & Semel, E.M. _Language assessment and intervention_. Columbus, OH: Charles E. Merrill Publishing Co., 1980.

Wiig, E.H. & Semel, E.M. _Language disabilities in children and adolescents_. Columbus, OH: Charles E. Merrill Publishing Company, 1976.

Wilkinson, A., Stratta, L. & Dudley, P. School council oracy project. In: _The quality of listening_. London: Macmillan Education, 1974.

Williams, S.S. Building listener accountability. _The Speech Teacher_, 1974, 23, 53-56.

Willis, V. & Garrison, M., Jr. Spoken language abilities of educable mentally retarded normal adolescents. _Psychological reports_, 1970, 26, 696-698.

Wilt, M. A study of teacher awareness of listening as a factor in elementary education. Journal of Educational Research, April 1950, 43.

Wolvin, A. & Coakley, C. Listening. Dubuque, IA: W.C. Brown Company Publishers, 1982.

Wood, B. Development of functional communication competencies: Grades 7-12. Urbana, IL: Clearinghouse on Reading and Communication Skills, 1977.

Woodcock, R. & Johnson, M.B. Woodcock-Johnson psycho-educational battery. Bingham, MA: Teaching Resources, 1977.

Work, R., Ehren, B., DeWitt, J., Bacoats, G. Are there really language disorders in the secondary school population? Paper presented at American Speech-Language-Hearing Association Convention in Toronto, Ontario, Canada, November 1982.

Worthley, W. Source book of language learning activities: Instructional strategies and methods. Boston, MA: Little, Brown & Co., Inc., 1978.

Wright, J., Norris, R. & Worsley, F. Concepts of communication unit #3: Communications. Niles, IL: Developmental Learning Materials, 1974.

Zemlin, W. Speech and hearing science, anatomy and physiology. Englewood Cliffs, NJ: Prentice-Hall, Inc., 1968.